SIX YE *and* COUNTING

Love, Leukemia, and the Long Road Onward

PETER GORDON

outskirts
press

This book is dedicated to all the wonderful people around the world who have registered to become marrow donors. Thousands of us blood cancer survivors are alive today only because we were able to receive a transplant from a matching donor among your ranks. We can literally say that we owe our lives to you!

To join these heroes, a simple cheek swab is all it takes - you may end up saving a life. For more information, please contact either of these perfectly-named organizations:

- Gift of Life (giftoflife.org)
- Be the Match (bethematch.org)

Thanks, and enjoy the story!

---Peter

TABLE OF CONTENTS

Part 1

INKLINGS

I still remember the tingle of the spring snow splattering against my face. It was spraying from RJ's skis, and I was right on his tail. It was mid-April. A bunch of us ski instructors were enjoying a season-ending play day at our neighboring ski area Wildcat. No lessons today – just a gaggle of middle-aged guys whooping and frolicking down the mountain like teenage boys. I carved a big arcing turn and shot ahead of the group. Suddenly a voice cried out from above: "Hold up! Here's the turnoff!" A local Wildcat instructor was showing us the way to a secret run down a snow-filled stream bed. I hit the brakes as hard as I could, but by the time I stopped, I was about a hundred feet below the others. "Hey Peter, you coming? We'll wait for ya." Normally a hundred foot sidestep up a gentle ski slope would be nothing for me, especially to join my buddies for an off-the-beaten-track run through the woods - the type of terrain I usually love. But for some reason, I didn't feel up to the climb. "No, you guys go ahead. I'll meet you at the bottom."

I picked up the phone. "Good morning, Peter Gordon."

"Hi Peter. This is Crystal from Mountain Medical."

"Oh, hi Crystal. How you doing?"

"Fine. I wanted to follow up from your exam yesterday. Your blood

1

test results just came back from the lab, and some of the numbers seem a little off. It's probably nothing – maybe the machine wasn't calibrated properly. But just to be sure, would you mind coming back in for another blood test?"

"Sure, no problem. Can I swing by tomorrow morning sometime?"

"How about 9:00 am?"

"That's perfect. See you then."

———◦———

Mary Ann was at her Book Club meeting with several neighbors from the resort where we lived. As part of the usual chit-chat among the ladies, she mentioned that she was a bit worried about my two recent blood tests, especially now that they were sending me to a hematologist for further testing. Every woman in the group offered some sort of reassuring phrase: "Oh, I'm sure it's nothing... The labs make mistakes all the time... Peter's such a strong healthy guy... I'm sure he'll be fine," etc. Every woman, that is, except our neighbor Peg - a retired nurse, a real no-nonsense type. Peg didn't say a word, but for a split second she caught Mary Ann's eye and gave her a fleeting glance – a glance of concern. In that instant (as I only found out months later), Mary Ann first knew...

———◦———

It was a beautiful spring morning as I sauntered into the Littleton Hospital. My mind was on my hike that afternoon, wondering how the footing would be now that the snow was melting. A cheerful elderly volunteer greeted me at the information desk – she was wearing a bright red vest with buttons all over it, like a Walmart greeter. I told her I was there to follow up on some blood tests and I was looking for a Dr. Diener. "Oh yes, he's in the oncology clinic, down the hall, third door on the right." *Oncology? I thought he was a hematologist. Hmmm...*

As I entered the clinic, the receptionist welcomed me warmly - unusually so for a medical office. What a friendly place, I thought, as I settled into my seat in the waiting area. I noticed they had a little garden outside the waiting room window, its plants just starting to come to life after the long New Hampshire winter. What a nice touch. I glanced around at the brightly colored posters on the wall and brochures in the display rack. Posters with beautiful photos of flowers and waterfalls and rays of sunshine, and little sayings about positive attitudes and compassion and love; brochures about support groups and caregiver counseling and living wills and - oh my god - hospice care! A shiver swept through me, and I felt my world shift.

———○———

I'm lying on my stomach on the examining table, my pants pulled down a bit to expose my hip. Dr. Diener apologizes in advance for what some patients find to be a very uncomfortable procedure. He calmly explains exactly how he's going to extract the bone marrow sample from my hip bone, step by step. I find this helpful. The nurse rubs a freezing antiseptic swab across the entry spot. The cold suddenly dissolves into searing heat as injections of painkiller burn under my skin. Doc asks if the spot's numb. I catch a glimpse of a sleek rod with a sharp little thing on the end and a handle on top. The nurse takes hold of my hand. Diener pushes the tool into my backside. Hardly any pain as it pierces the skin, then I feel an odd little bump as it hits bone. He cautions me this may be uncomfortable. I feel the tool twisting and grinding into my hip, the pressure pushing me down into the cushion on the table. Not too painful as long as I stay relaxed and breathe. More bothersome are the vibrations and squeaks as he grinds away. Diener asks if I'm OK. Doing fine, I say. Here comes the tough part, he says, again almost apologetically. Suddenly I think I feel the tool break through the bone into the soft marrow chamber inside. A different kind of feeling like nothing I've ever experienced - a strange tingling pulsating burn deep inside. Again, breathing helps. Diener asks again how I'm doing. I say OK. He says he's almost done, then suddenly he's out. As the nurse whisks away the tools and dressings, out of the corner of my eye I notice what looks like a little vial – I assume it contains my bone marrow sample. They patch me up with a small dressing. I hitch up my pants and hop up off the table. They say I handled it unusually well.

This is not your run-of-the-mill blood test. The bone marrow Dr. Diener has extracted from my hip will be sent to a special lab for biopsy – a much deeper, more complex analysis than the regular blood tests I've had so far. The analysis will take a week. I schedule a follow-up appointment with Diener to review the results, then I head home...

I remember walking back to my car that day, weaving through the puddles from the melting snow piles in the hospital parking lot, wondering about that little vial and what its contents would reveal. I knew a lot was at stake. I'm not sure if Mary Ann or I or anyone had as yet even given voice to the "C" word, but it was certainly lurking in our minds, deep below the surface, more menacing in the unspoken recesses of our fears than out in the open.

Yes, I knew the contents of that vial would determine a lot. But now, as I reflect back on it years later, I realize I didn't have a clue about all it really contained. Bone marrow is like a super-fertile breeding ground for new blood cells – in many ways, even a source of life itself. Well, the marrow sample in that little vial would become the source of an unimagined journey, taking me to places I never dreamed of. It would chart a course not only for my next few years, but for the rest of my life. It would change my world, and lead me into the depths of my own soul. And it would be the wellspring of a deeper love than I had ever imagined possible...

But I'm not thinking about any of that as I leave the hospital that morning in the spring of 2008. All I know is that little vial contains the answer to why my blood counts have gone haywire lately. It'll turn uncertainty into concrete knowledge, and waiting into tangible action steps, whatever they may be. And that's good enough for me.

I tuck away my thoughts about the biopsy results into a little compartment in the back of my mind. My appointment with Dr. Diener is a week away, so I turn off that switch and refocus on the moment. I'm already packed and prepared for my business trip to New York the next morning, so I'm going to reward myself with an afternoon hike. It'll be great to get out into the warm spring air, and start transitioning those leg muscles from skiing to hiking season. I hop across the last of the puddles, step into my car, and head home.

INKLINGS

Despite a sore backside, lots of mud and slush on the trail, and a bit more huffing and puffing than usual, my hike that afternoon turns out to be wonderful.

Part 2

THE BACK STORY

efore I bring you to my meeting with Dr. Diener in a week, I'd like to pause here to fill you in on the background, and give you some context. In particular, you may be wondering what's all this about being a ski instructor and living with someone named Mary Ann in a New Hampshire mountain resort? How in the world did I end up there?

Well, the short answer is that it was an example of how a difficult loss can transform into something unexpectedly good. A rebirth of sorts.

For a longer answer, I'd like to tell you the story of how I got to that point. This will set the stage for everything that follows. But it's far more than just background. It's also like an "overture," offering glimpses of many issues to come: a brush with cancer, other health scares, relationships, family, loss, rebuilding, self-discovery. A story that not only previewed many of the challenges I would face, but also helped me prepare for them.

At least I think that's why it's a worthwhile prelude. On the other hand, maybe it's just something I want to get out there. Who knows. Anyway, here's the back story. It unfolds over the next forty pages or so. It's quite a tale - I hope you enjoy it.

So how did I end up being a ski instructor living in a mountain resort with a woman named Mary Ann?

6

The mountain home dream comes true

After 41 years of bachelorhood, I married my first wife back in 1995. We settled in Lincoln, Massachusetts, a pleasant, mostly rural town outside of Boston. She was a Human Resources manager, and I was a corporate trainer. She commuted to her company's office in nearby Cambridge every day; I had a little office at home, and typically traveled to various US cities a few days each week to deliver training workshops.

While we were successful in our careers, we also loved outdoor recreation. After work we'd go jogging, swimming, bicycling, canoeing - you name it. On weekends, we'd often head up to the northern New England mountains to hike, camp, or ski. Our neighbors made good-natured fun of the way we were always loading our car with various types of sports gear, teasing us that our active lifestyle was "right out of a catalog." I guess they had a point – we were sort of recreation nuts. But frankly, I was thrilled to have finally found a partner with whom I could share my passion for the great outdoors.

My wife was more than just a sports companion, however. I was drawn to her calm, pleasant manner; to the softness of her voice; to the kindness in her heart, especially toward animals, kids, and the elderly; to her diligence and professionalism at work; to the harmonious way we did chores together - indeed virtually everything together. We just seemed to get along. Some even called us "the perfect couple" in those early years.

Our home was constantly bustling with whiffle-ball games and dinner parties and dogs. We both had families nearby, so we were always visiting with relatives and taking care of nieces and nephews. I shared Red Sox season tickets, and we spent many fun evenings at Fenway Park cheering for our local baseball heroes. We rehabbed much of our home. We planted gardens. We took hundred-mile bike rides. We went to shows. Our energy was boundless, and our life around Lincoln was abuzz.

Even so, we felt an increasingly strong pull from the mountains to our north. We loved our weekend getaways up there, though constantly packing and unpacking all that gear started to become a chore.

We longed to be settled in a mountain "base camp" somewhere, so we decided to look for a place of our own.

While a second home may have once seemed like an extravagant dream, it was now looking increasingly doable. We were both making decent incomes, and we had no kids (or college tuitions). We were able to put away some savings, much of which I invested in an aggressive mutual fund specializing in those late 90's dotcom companies. Remember them? Well the fund kept appreciating at a staggering rate - every month I'd open my statement and shake my head in amazement. I knew this bonanza wouldn't last. But if we played our cards right, it just might pay for our vacation home.

After exploring all over northern New England, we focused on Bretton Woods, New Hampshire. It was far enough north to be beyond the weekend hordes from greater Boston, but still within reach. The setting was spectacular, with the Presidential Range as a backdrop and the White Mountain National Forest all around. We liked that it was an established resort, anchored by the iconic Mt. Washington Hotel. It had a ski area, tennis courts, biking and cross-country trails, a couple restaurants, a little store, and a small community of condo owners. All nestled together in a remote mountain valley. A four-season getaway. This was the place.

A nice townhouse soon came on the market – plenty of room, move-in condition, a private hillside setting, and a spectacular view. We decided to jump on it. So in early March, 2000, I cashed out of the mutual fund, and used the proceeds to pay for our new mountain condo. Our dream had become a reality!

Interestingly, a few days after we closed on our purchase, the NASDAQ market collapsed and the dotcom stock bubble burst. I guess that turned out to be a fortunate bit of good timing for us! (In hindsight, however, also an ominous reminder that you can't take anything for granted, be it a stock market surge, good health, or for that matter, a marriage.)

I remember our excitement arriving those first few Friday evenings, opening the door and pinching ourselves that this was actually our own place! We had a blast setting up our mountain retreat. We searched local antique stores for furniture and knick-knacks. My wife made curtains and added mountain-themed decor touches. I built a gear closet, with our skis and snowshoes and backpacks all arranged just so. And of course, we got out and explored our new ski area during the last weeks of the season – I was especially thrilled to discover so many hidden runs through the woods.

The melting snow soon revealed more surprises about our mountain world: hiking and biking trails, river gorges and waterfalls, fields of wildflowers, the back verandah over at the hotel, a great old-time summer theater in nearby Bethlehem. Summer gave way to spectacular fall foliage, followed by the excitement of the first new snow on the Presidential Range, and then the depths of a snowy winter. It was an amazing place to experience the richness of the four seasons in all their glory. That first year we ended up going 46 out of 52 weekends!

The drives up and back became a regular part of our routine, one of the rhythms of our life. Average driving time was a little over two and a half hours, a bit less if we flirted with a speeding ticket (which we never got, as we learned all the state cops' favorite hiding places), and often more on busy weekends.

But no matter how long the drive took, or how stressful the traffic-clogged crawl out of greater Boston was, as soon as you'd pull into the parking lot and turn off the motor, that would all dissolve away. The second you step out of the car and feel the crisp cool air, and you see the pink alpenglow on the Presidential peaks, or the dazzling stars and Milky Way splashed across the sky horizon to horizon, and you hear that mesmerizing quiet, not an empty sterile quiet devoid of sound, but an even deeper and more soothing quiet, a quiet softened by the distant sounds of the rushing river, or the breezes drifting over the mountain ridges, or forlorn calls from wildlife deep in the forest, in that very second you feel the fibers of your body loosen, and you exhale the tension and hurried pace and mental clutter from the work week - even if you didn't realize you had it until you feel it dissipate - and as you breathe back in, you feel the mountain air cleansing your mind and recharging your soul. You haven't even reached the front door yet, and you're already transformed. The rest of the weekend is gravy.

Over the next few years, we shuttled back and forth between our two homes, our two worlds. Our Bretton Woods townhouse had lots of room, and the place was often filled with visitors, including the occasional dog or two. As you can probably imagine, we were always on the go somewhere in our mountain playground. And after a day outdoors, what a great place to relax - sipping a warm drink in front of the fireplace, or hanging out on the deck, watching the sunset over the mountains, then the incredible stars. Our mountain getaway turned out to be everything I'd dreamed of, and more.

My wife was exceptionally strong and fit. Whether cycling up a mountain pass or cross-country skiing on a backcountry trail, she always seemed to glide along effortlessly, often smiling, never a sign of strain on her face. She never appeared to struggle. Except once.

After several years at Bretton Woods, we'd climbed most of the mountains around our valley, many of them repeatedly. One that we'd never done, however, was Mt. Willey, a spectacular peak rising steeply for about 3,000 vertical feet, its summit visible right from our dining room table. One day we decided to give it a try. About halfway up, I noticed my wife's pace was unusually slow, and for once she didn't have that effortless demeanor. Something was wrong. She said she didn't feel well and asked if we could go back down, almost apologizing. No problem at all, I said. (That's a mountaineering ethic I've always admired – there's absolutely no shame in turning around when things aren't right. Mountains and machismo don't mix.) We headed back down to the condo and took it easy for the rest of the weekend.

A few weeks later, I was on a business trip in California that kept me out there over the weekend. When I called my wife in Bretton Woods, she told me that she'd just returned from Mt. Willey – she'd gone back up there and climbed it on her own! I was impressed and proud. When I came home, I told her I'd honor her accomplishment by never climbing Mt. Willey myself. I'd always consider it to be *her* peak, something special to keep as her own. I thought that was a nice gesture.

Dissolution and displacement

Looking back, I can't put my finger on exactly when it started. Who knows, maybe it had been happening for years, hidden somewhere deep below the surface, festering, metastasizing, obscured by our vigorous lifestyle, or my rose-colored optimism, or her soft voice and calm smile. But I started noticing it somewhere around 2003. I sensed things seemed to be cooling between us, and she was drawing away.

Nothing dramatic or sudden. No huge blow-ups or traumas. While we did seem to have more little spats (usually over things that seemed relatively minor to me), I wrote those off to the squabbling typical of most couples as they grow older together. More subtle, but much more telling to me, was how those moments of affection, connection, and playfulness from our earlier years had somehow withered away. She just seemed more distant.

I couldn't get a handle on what was going on. Was she OK? Was it me? Was it something else? Who knows? We didn't really talk about it. Maybe that was part of the problem.

I wondered if the recent changes in our work lives might have been throwing our rhythms off. My corporate training was transitioning to more of a freelance role; I'd also started teaching part-time at a nearby college, which I loved. My wife's job was evolving too, broadening beyond HR into property management as she led her company through a major relocation. She was spending increasingly long hours at work, searching for new office space and then managing the complex moving process.

But all that seemed fine with me – it's healthy to keep reinventing your work life with new challenges. No, something else was going on. It was a strange, unsettled time, rolling along with our ever-active life while sensing a growing hollowness on the inside.

And then, right in the middle of this period, she came down with breast cancer.

Talk about knocking your life out of its rhythms! Ours became unhinged. Ironically, however, this also gave a sense of purpose to all the uncertainty. I remember shifting gears immediately, tucking away the worry about our relationship into one of those mental compartments, and focusing on helping my wife through her cancer.

Only problem was, I didn't really know what to do. I defaulted to my usual role of trying to be the "good husband," taking care of the tangible things, giving her rides, doing a little extra around the house, cooking, cleaning, whatever. Sure, we talked about appointments and test results and the like, but we didn't talk at that deeper level where you just spill out your inner feelings. She never opened up about what she really needed from me to help her through her cancer, and frankly, it never dawned on me to ask. I was just wallowing around in the world of task management, vaguely frustrated that I couldn't connect with my wife more deeply.

Why did she seem so aloof? Was this a normal side effect of cancer? Why did I feel so held at arm's length? Do all cancer spouses experience this? I felt more like a roommate than a partner, more like an attendant than a caregiver. No, that's not exactly correct; in hindsight, I realize that the concept of being a "caregiver" - not just the word but the role, the skill, the art - wasn't even on my radar. I was just a husband struggling to do the right thing for an increasingly distant wife, and I didn't have a clue...

Well it turned out they caught the cancer in time. She did require a series of radiation treatments to prevent it from recurring, and for several weeks I took her to her appointments. I'll always remember the atmosphere in the radiation clinic waiting area. This was not your typical medical office, with everyone quietly immersed in their People magazines and smartphones. No, quite the opposite. I was struck by the warm camaraderie among the "regulars" there for their treatments, my wife included. I was surprised by the light-hearted chit-chat, the jokes, the goodwill - amazed how such an awful disease can bond a group of strangers, and transform a hospital waiting room into a happy place. Although of course I didn't realize it at the time, this was a preview of something I'd experience years later.

By all reports, my wife's cancer was soon under control and her prognosis was optimistic. Always on the pragmatic side, I was ready to refocus on getting our life back to normal. But my wife still seemed withdrawn, even more so than before. Her late hours at work continued. She also started spending more and more time with a yoga group. I wondered if the cancer had somehow changed her, driven her more into her own private world. Maybe recovering from cancer was a longer, more complex process than I'd thought, and she needed these refuges as part of her healing. After all, what could be better for her body and spirit than yoga? Not unlike the thinking behind my Mt. Willey gesture, I figured a little space might be good for her, and good for us.

But all we ended up doing with that space was drifting further apart in it, like planets moving out of the gravitational pull that holds them together. I felt nine years of marriage slipping away, going ice cold, and I didn't know how to bring it back.

We were cruising down from Bretton Woods one Sunday evening during the summer of 2004, when out of the blue she blurted out that she wanted a divorce. Though I wasn't totally surprised, it still hit me like a brick. I guess it was hearing the "D" word - divorce was something that happened to *other* people. It was one of those moments when, in just a few seconds and a few words, you know your whole life has changed. There would be more.

I didn't really fight it. I accepted that the fire had gone out, and all the reasoning and arguing and pleading in the world wouldn't rekindle it. What kept grating on me, though, was that I could never get a clear answer why. Sometimes she'd say something about "control." Other times she'd mention relatively small incidents from the past - little quarrels we'd had or things I'd said. The reasons kept changing. The only constant was that none seemed significant enough to toss away nine years of what had seemed like a pretty good marriage overall. It was painful enough facing that loss. What made it even harder was the vagueness, the uncertainty, the wavering reasons floating from one thing to another, with no substance, like grasping at clouds.

That August I had a work trip lined up at a nice conference resort in Arizona. When making my travel plans, I tacked on a few extra days hoping my wife would come along. She could enjoy relaxing at the resort while I was conducting my workshops, and then we'd take a road trip through the spectacular Southwest. I was hoping the change of scenery might revive things between us. It was my last gasp attempt to rescue our marriage. She said no.

I ended up taking that road trip alone. The Southwestern scenery was beautiful, the open-road adventure reviving nostalgic memories of a more free-spirited era. But it also brought back something else from the past, something I thought had been eradicated forever: that old, aching loneliness.

I remember wading up the narrow slot canyon at Zion National Park, mesmerized by the shafts of sunlight and reflections shimmering across the vertical walls above. It reminded me of those carnival funhouse mirrors that distort everything. Yes, my life was all scrambled. I trudged up the shallow stream for miles, lost in thought, the canyon walls narrowing to barely more than arms-length width. Suddenly it hit me that I hadn't seen another person for hours. I felt a little shudder of fear, then turned back.

I strolled through the magnificent Teddy Roosevelt-era hotel at the Grand Canyon, admiring the huge beams and massive stone fireplace and antlered animal heads on the walls. I walked into the restaurant and asked for a table for one. It reminded me of that Woody Allen movie where he does the same thing, and suddenly all the other diners halt their conversations and stare while a spotlight shines on him walking alone to his table. I chuckled to myself, but it only masked a deeper fear: The fear of going backward, back to so many years of searching, hoping, longing - back to the emptiness I thought I'd left behind forever on that joyous day I finally got married at age 41 - and now at 50 facing the dread of having to go back there again.

Sitting on a cliff perched over the Grand Canyon is a great place to think – for some reason, the vastness of the setting helps you explore more deeply inside your own self. I realized I'd been naive to think that just going on a trip together would revive our relationship. I reflected on my own "coulda's:" Maybe I could've been a better listener; maybe

I could've been less set in my ways; maybe I could've been more ambitious or accomplished. But even so, these still didn't seem to add up to the point where she'd just want to walk away. The math didn't feel right.

I wondered if our hyper-active lifestyle had been a diversion that kept us from the deep conversations and nurturing a relationship requires. Or maybe it was a veneer, a shiny surface masking some sort of decay underneath.

In any case, I returned from the Southwest resigned to accept the loss, stop worrying about its cause, and start moving ahead.

Compared to the horror stories you hear about divorcing couples fighting over kids, finances, furniture, and so on, ours had little drama. We decided she'd keep the place in Lincoln so she could keep commuting to her job. I'd take the condo up in Bretton Woods, using that as my home base, and flying off to my corporate training gigs from the Manchester, NH airport.

As that summer of 2004 faded, we stayed busy with work and continued weekend trips up to Bretton Woods. In a bizarre, almost surreal paradox, we kept enjoying many of our usual activities together up there, while using the drives back and forth to transport our stuff to each home in preparation for our impending split. Every so often, I'd check to see if she still wanted to go through with it, or if she could give me a clearer understanding of the reasons why. Her reasons kept wavering, but she remained resolute in her decision to leave. Her demeanor was always calm, pleasant, with no sign of strain - just like out on those cross-country ski trails.

September 11th, 2004, was a perfect day for hiking – clear and crisp, with the foliage starting to change colors. That morning at breakfast, my wife insisted that we take separate hikes. Separate hikes! Maybe it was her way of signaling the end of things, marking her independence – she didn't explain why. It was as if we were communicating through the language of our hikes rather than through words. In any case, it hurt.

In the White Mountains of New Hampshire, they have a great tradition to honor those who died in the September 11th terrorist attacks: There are 48 peaks over 4,000 feet high, and every September 11th, various volunteer groups carry a large American flag to the summit of every one of them. That day I climbed Mt. Jackson, elevation 4,052 feet. From the rocky summit I looked down on our resort village clustered toy-like way below. I borrowed some binoculars and spotted several American flags on nearby peaks – a very moving sight. I scanned across the jagged ridges of the Presidential Range and made out the summit of Mt. Jefferson several miles away. My wife was up there somewhere. As the large American flag flapped in the breeze above me, the sadness of that memorial, the majesty of the mountains, and the emptiness of the moment swirled together in a way I'll never forget.

When I got back to the condo, the pain had congealed into purpose. Though my wife had already taken most of her clothes down to Lincoln, her sports equipment remained. It was time. I opened the gear closet and removed her downhill and cross-county skis, poles, snowshoes, hiking gear, and whatnot, and stacked it against the wall alongside the path to the parking lot. For some reason, I lined up everything in perfect order, sequentially by height, equally spaced, perfectly parallel. I'm not sure why. On one hand, I'm sort of a compulsive neatnick - I'm one of those types who always sorts the bills in my wallet by denomination and faces them all the same way. But maybe it was more than that. Could it have been my own little passive aggressive response to the separate hikes? To the whole break-up? Who knows?

When my wife saw her gear spread out along the wall, her calm demeanor finally cracked. It was the only time during our separation process that I saw her cry. We packed the last of her stuff into the car and drove down to Lincoln together. She would never be back.

A couple days later, the home I'd owned and shared for almost ten years was empty of me. I had one last carload packed up, and it was time to leave Lincoln for the last time. I don't recall anything about my departure, or saying goodbye, or anything...

...Funny, though - I do remember arriving up in Bretton Woods a few hours later that evening. The usual welcoming sensations greeted me as I turned off the engine and stepped out of the car: the crisp air, the soothing quiet, the spectacular stars - all very familiar. But something was different. As I heard the leaves scratching across the parking lot in the cool breeze, a little shiver rippled through me. I realized this wasn't my getaway place anymore – it was my home.

Bridging the emptiness

The bedroom shades slide open, the stairs creak under my footsteps, the coffee maker chugs and hisses, the spoon clinks against the cup as I stir in the milk and sugar. The sounds echo through the empty house as if they're coming from someone else. I feel like a stranger in my own place. It's day one.

I start unpacking my Lincoln clothes, strategizing how to reposition everything in the closet. My dress clothes seem so foreign mixing in with all my casual stuff. At least there's a lot of empty space in the closet now. Empty space... The ache starts welling up from deep inside, like when you feel the first hint of nausea coming on and you try to calm it back down. I refocus on hanging my ties in perfect order of color gradation, from yellows to reds to blues. The ache subsides.

I dump out a box of my bathroom supplies from Lincoln. There's that cute little Gumby-shaped bar of soap from Disney World. Happy times at Disney... The ache wells up again. I calm it down by sorting razor blades and tooth brushes.

Driving down to our little village of Twin Mountain, I notice the bright foliage colors along the banks of the Ammonoosuc River. There's that bend in the river where we held hands and hopped across the smoothly rounded rocks and tossed sticks into the icy water and the dog would dive in afterward, scampering back up the bank with the stick in its mouth, tail wagging, eager for more, shaking itself off, spraying us with cold water and warm laughter... Here it comes again - a queasy, dizzying wave. Breathe. Refocus. Review the plan for my errands in town: Post Office, Town Hall, car registration, inspection sticker, register to vote…

———◈———

And so it went that fall. Little triggers everywhere - sometimes a place, sometimes a song, sometimes a random memory or fleeting thought – and then the pain would well up and envelop me. My only refuge was absorbing myself in the present, one task at a time, no matter how mundane, filling the emptiness and warding off the past. The future didn't exist.

One such refuge was my corporate training work. When I was away in another city, absorbed in my workshop, that gave me purpose and focus. Even if I'd delivered the program a hundred times before, for those learners in the room it was new, and I'd immerse myself into the experience from their perspective. That helped – it gave me eight hours' escape. Fortunately, the economy was doing well, and I had lots of work booked.

Weekends would bring an influx of people to the resort and a different type of refuge: hanging out with neighbors. Typical chat would include our hiking exploits, favorite microbrews, the latest resort gossip, and always the most burning question of all: When's the snow gonna start falling? Once in a while, there'd be an awkward moment when they'd ask where my wife was. Fortunately, the awkwardness was fleeting, as everyone accepted things with barely a hitch and moved on. My neighbors were great.

But just like the receding tide, on Sunday afternoons the place would empty out. Remember that mountain quiet I used to find so soothing? Well now it was more unsettling, leaving me feeling alone and exposed.

I tried playing little "positivity" games in my mind: For every aspect of my new life, I'd ask myself what's different, what's better? For example, now a New Hampshire resident, I no longer had to pay state income taxes – that was excellent. I set up a little office with a spectacular view of the ski trails right from my desk – how many people get a view like that from their workplace? My new license plates had a picture of a moose – how cool! And one more thing about those license plates: They were emblazoned with the quirky NH state motto "Live Free or Die." Sort of a harsh edge to it, but I got a kick out of it.

All these little refuges and positive thoughts helped, but they gave only temporary and superficial relief, like putting lip balm over chapped lips. The pain was always lurking below, and every now and then it would bubble up, with no warning, no pattern, totally unpredictable - that was the hardest part.

Another type of refuge that autumn was baseball. Yes, baseball - in particular, the Boston Red Sox. I guess there's something therapeutic about getting swept away in a story outside your own world; it's like the escape you get from a good movie, except a baseball pennant race is a longer drama, extending for weeks. And as it turned out for me that fall, baseball ended up being far more than just an escape.

The Red Sox games would fill up my evenings. Most nights would find me gazing intently at the TV, watching every pitch, analyzing every swing, transported into another world for three hours. Other times, I'd head down to the local watering hole Fabyan's to grab a burger and beer. It was a sanctuary that fall, much like the bar in Cheers. No matter who'd belly up to the bar, whether local or tourist, you'd always end up chatting about the Sox game on the TV.

The Red Sox had gone 86 years without a World Series win – so many close calls, so many dashed hopes, heartache woven into the fabric of New England culture. But in the fall of 2004, hopes were high that this might be the year.

There was something special about that Red Sox team – not just their talent on the field, but something about their wacky cast of characters and zany demeanor. I was captivated by the way they managed to stay loose, cope with the ups and downs, make great comebacks. How they shifted so smoothly between intensity and light-heartedness. There's so much more to making it through a long baseball season than just the plays on the field - the intangibles matter.

Baseball intertwined with family in a special way that fall. The Red

Sox made the playoffs, and I had tickets to a couple post-season games. Without my wife, now I could invite others. So I took my brother Larry to one of the first-round playoff games against the Angels. The Red Sox were one win away from sweeping the series. It was an agonizing game, with the Sox jumping out to a big lead, only to lose it in the late innings. The old familiar worry and self-doubt of Sox fans started creeping in. Then in the bottom of the tenth inning, David Ortiz hit a monster walk-off home run to end the game and the series. Fenway went absolutely nuts. The jubilant crowd spilled out on the streets, sweeping us along, whoops of joy everywhere, car horns blaring. We joined right in with the celebration. I'll always remember my brother Larry – normally on the reserved side - walking down the sidewalk high-fiving total strangers. That was a rare and priceless sight!

I knew the jubilation on that sidewalk would be a short-lived rush, but that didn't matter – I hadn't laughed or celebrated or felt unabashed joy in a long time.

The next series was against the archrival New York Yankees. Unfortunately the Red Sox lost the first three games. Lose four and you're out. All the optimism was seeping away, drop by drop. I was driving in my car barely listening to game four with half an ear, as I'd pretty much given up by then. Down three games to zero, the Sox were two runs behind, with two outs in the ninth inning, bases empty, and they were facing Mariano Rivera, the greatest relief pitcher in history. You can't get any closer to all hope being lost than that. But then Dave Roberts got on base and, in a gutsy and audacious move, stole second. Suddenly that dying ember flickered back to life, igniting the faintest hope. For some reason, I pulled the car over to the side of the road and listened to the rest of the game from there. Something told me the Sox actually had a chance.

Sure enough, they came back to win that game. Then they clawed their way back to win the next two games as well, evening the series at 3-3. I found myself at my brother Larry's house in Concord for the decisive seventh game. When the Red Sox won, it was quite the opposite of the sidewalk delirium we'd shared outside Fenway Park a couple weeks earlier. Larry, his son Sam, and I just sat there in stunned silence, unable to put words to the significance of the amazing comeback we'd just witnessed – probably the greatest in sports history. I remember thinking at the time about what a powerful lesson those Red Sox gave about persistence, optimism, never giving up.

The Red Sox entered the World Series against the St. Louis Cardinals. Two teams rich in history and tradition - that's when baseball is at its best. My father Bob used to tell stories about the Red Sox of his era, featuring the great Ted Williams, playing the Cardinals in the 1946 World Series, and coming so close, losing game seven in a heartbreaker. I loved his baseball stories from the old days. Baseball was one place we always found common ground.

Then there was that magical season of 1967, when the "Impossible Dream" Red Sox made it to the World Series, again against St. Louis. I remember a few of us 9th graders skipping class, hiding in the boys' locker room, huddled around a scratchy transistor radio listening to our Sox battle the Cardinals and their fearsome pitcher Bob Gibson. Again, they lost in seven games – oh so close.

And now here we were 37 years later, once again facing St. Louis in the World Series. And guess who had a pair of tickets! I could have sold them for thousands. But there was no way I was going to miss that game, and there was no hesitation about whom to invite: How could it be anyone other than my father? In 1961, he'd taken me to my first game at Fenway, against the legendary Mantle-and-Maris Yankees no less. (How can any kid ever forget their first walk up that dark ballpark tunnel, then seeing the dazzling green field burst into view?) And now here we were at the World Series, live and in person – what an honor to make it my treat this time.

Old Fenway was magnificent that night, dressed up in American flag bunting. James Taylor sang the national anthem - one of the most beautiful versions of that song I've ever heard. Even gruff, old-school Bob said he liked it. The Sox ended up winning. It turned out to be the famous game in which Curt Shilling pitched through the pain of recent ankle surgery, with the blood still leaking from the incision and staining his sock red. You could see the bloody sock from our seats - one of those iconic images that will live on in sports lore forever.

Sharing that game with my father was one of the highlights of my life, and I don't just mean sports highlights.

The aptly named Red Sox kept their momentum going through the rest of the series, and they had a 3-0 lead, on the brink of "reversing the curse" and finally winning the World Series for the first time in 86 years. I was watching with my brother Eric and his family in Lexington. Red Sox Nation was tuned in, fingers crossed, optimistic but on edge – all too familiar with heartbreak.

When the ball went to first for the final out, probably everybody in New England jumped up and screamed. We sure did! I'll always remember Eric and Marcia and Julia and Ben leaping up, arms outstretched, seeming to hang in the air like a mobile, floating with joy and disbelief. It was an amazing feeling of lightness, as if a heavy burden had suddenly dissolved.

Once I finally sat down, a different type of feeling surged through me. I put my hands over my face, ran into the bathroom, buckled to my knees in front of the toilet, and – no, it's not what you think – I propped my elbows on the toilet, buried my face in my hands, and just exploded in tears, sobs, wails. Cried like I'd never cried before. All the pain of losing my marriage and our happy times at Fenway just combusted inside me, spewing out uncontrollably, volcano-like. I tried my best to muffle the sounds.

I now realize that all those little refuges and optimistic mind-games had been only superficial anesthesia, suppressing, but not releasing, the pain deep inside. How ironic that it took a wonderfully happy event to let it all out. I guess that's the way the grieving and healing process works – you can't expect everything to be logical.

Anyway, that night was a turning point for me. The pain of my lost marriage started to ebb, but the glow of the Red Sox victory remained. It was Halloween, October 31, 2004.

A few weeks later I was in Boston with my family for Thanksgiving – my first as a single guy in ten years. I was feeling OK, maybe still a bit empty and numb. Mostly I was just self-conscious about being alone. I wondered if the others were looking at me funny. My discomfort must have shown.

At a break in the meal, my mother Nancy pulled me aside. She put her hand on my shoulder, looked me in the eye, and handed me a ring my father had given her many years before – a spectacular jade ring he bought in Singapore. "I'd like you to have this ring. Do with it whatever you will," she said. "And I want you to know that you're going to find more happiness in your life than you ever imagined. I just know it. I guarantee it." As you'll see in this story, I'm not much for hollow words of encouragement – I generally prefer substance. But at that moment, I somehow felt that my mother's words did have meaning. For some reason, I really believed her. Suddenly my hopes flickered back to life, much like when Dave Roberts stole that base.

Nancy's words gave me something to latch on to. They transplanted the future back into me. That little bit of Thanksgiving-day encouragement was one of the best (of many) gifts she ever gave me. And as mothers usually are when they tell their kids stuff, she sure turned out to be right.

Rebuilding steps

So that's how I ended up living in a mountain resort – in a nutshell, I got divorced, moved into the ski house, and built a new life from there. But there's more to the story, especially the "rebirth" part I mentioned earlier.

I think I've learned a few lessons about healing during my long journey. One of them is managing an apparent paradox: On one hand, an essential ingredient in healing is simply time; you have to be patient and allow the process to play out over its course – you have to just ride it through. On the other hand, you can't always be passive; sometimes it takes a little initiative here and there to nudge the healing process along.

I haven't always been a good initiative taker throughout my life. But for some reason, while riding through the healing process that fall, I took four action steps that ended up making a huge difference. A difference not only in recovering from my divorce, but also in helping me through much greater challenges to come.

The first was an impulse decision one day to walk over to the ski area and apply for a part-time job as a ski instructor. I'd always been a pretty good skier, with what everyone called "good form." Also, I was an educator by trade, with many years of teaching and coaching experience. So I figured I might have a knack for ski instructing. I knew there wasn't much money in it, but it would fill my weekends, get me more connected with people around our resort, and hell, I'd even get a free ski pass – a most valuable perk!

Well that turned out to be one of the greatest moves I ever made. I ended up making all sorts of friends, not only fellow instructors, but other employees, homeowners, resort guests, etc. That winter would be the first of many fun, rewarding seasons on the slopes. I loved working with our guests, not just to improve their skiing technique, but also to boost their confidence and joy. I also got a kick out of our own instructor training clinics - it was a bit humbling to realize my own skiing needed some tweaking, but I enjoyed the ongoing learning. And about the low pay – well, when every once in a while I'd get a $20 tip, I felt as if I'd won the lottery!

Another action step I took was to join several homeowner association committees. One of my specialties became grounds and tree maintenance, which was a very big issue for our condo village clustered on a forested mountainside. I also got involved organizing community clean-ups and similar events. Community service turned out to be very therapeutic, as it pulled me out of my own little world and broadened my perspective to larger issues of the common good. It also helped establish a groundwork for what would become a rich social life and, eventually, an incredible support network.

A third step I took that fall was to commit to a personal goal: Remember those 48 mountain peaks in New Hampshire over 4,000 high? Well I decided to climb them all. This was a common objective among hard-core New England hikers - to become a member of the "4,000-Footer Club." I figured I'd climbed about half of them over the years anyway, so completing the list would give me a goal to shoot for, along with some purpose and order to my otherwise unstructured free time. I'd never been much of a goal-oriented person, and I thought maybe it would do me some good.

So that fall I began my hiking quest. I was in pretty good shape to begin with, but before long I noticed that I was virtually skipping my way up and down the rugged terrain. I tore out the official 4,000-footer list from a hiking magazine, and put a little checkmark next to each peak I climbed. It was very motivating to see all those checkmarks piling up. Therapeutic too.

I didn't really have a systematic plan of attack - I'd choose my next peak based on the time required, the nature of the terrain, or whatever little whim came along. But I did make a clear decision on which peak I would tackle *last*: Remember Mt. Willey, the mountain I left unclimbed in honor of my wife? Well now that she was my ex-wife, it seemed fitting to complete my quest by climbing Mt. Willey last, reclaiming it for my own. I figured this would be a symbolic way to put closure on that chapter and move on. I found lots of power in that, and other symbols.

The fourth action I took was to start looking for a new companion. Although it would take a while to get over losing my marriage, part of me was eager to move ahead. After all, I'd enjoyed being married (at least up until the last couple years), and I started to long for it again. Plus, it was awfully cold and lonely up in those northern New Hampshire mountains. So I took someone's advice and joined Match. com, an online dating site. Having been in a relationship for over ten years, here I was at age 51, living in the middle of nowhere, re-entering the long-forgotten world of dating, and now pursuing it via the Internet no less!

Well I soon got the hang of how to use Match to create my online profile, and hopefully make it stand out. I noticed that many other profiles appeared to be little more than a generic list of "likes," often filled with standard clichés such as "I like walks on the beach," or "I like dining out," or "I seek someone who's honest and sincere." (Like, who doesn't?) Instead, I tried to reveal a little personality and humor. Among other things, I took a chance by mentioning that I always remembered to put the toilet seat down. Apparently that line worked.

My online dating adventure had much in common with my 4,000-footer hiking quest. Each was a major project that gave me purpose and direction. Each had an ultimate goal, though I wasn't obsessed with reaching it in a hurry. Instead, I decided to view both pursuits as meandering journeys. My hiking quest took me to scenic views, waterfalls, and beautiful places that I never would have seen otherwise. Same with my Match dates. I got glimpses into the lives of a kindergarten teacher, chamber of commerce director, artist, therapist, lawyer, potter, nurse, even an undertaker!

One of my earliest dates taught me something valuable. The dinner conversation flowed smoothly and I thought everything went well. However, as we left the restaurant, she told me she didn't want to pursue things further because she sensed I wasn't fully over my wife. That stung a bit at the time, but I soon realized she was right. The process of letting go and moving on is harder than you think, no matter how much you try to act like you're over it.

And how could I not mention my date with The Zen Guru? She was a therapist, meditation instructor, and spiritual counselor - all about helping others find calm and inner peace. Sounded intriguing - I could use some inner peace. So we met at a restaurant. About thirty seconds after we first sat down, she went into an absolute flip-out with the waiter about some innocuous thing – like whether a menu item was available in an entree sized portion or something like that. You should have heard her making a fuss, demanding to see the manager, actually yelling. The other diners turned toward us. I was cringing, sinking lower in my chair, trying to hide my face.

For the rest of the meal I tried to be civil, but in my mind I was thinking "*Get me the hell out of here ASAP.*" That date was painful, not least because I had to drive home 70 miles over mountain roads through a blizzard. (Glad I had a Subaru.) But in the end it was hilarious, adding one more memory to the richness of my dating adventure.

Some dates were a bit sad. I met several women who were perfectly nice, smart, interesting, etc. I could tell they were interested in me. But

26

I just didn't feel... ah... er... oh well, I think you know what I mean. That was hard; it hurt to let someone's hopes down. On the other hand, the same thing happened to me. You typically plan a first date by building in some "outs" along the way, and a couple times after one drink, they'd say they had to run. It was crystal clear what that meant in the language of dating. I never took it personally. In fact, I was relieved to skip that awkward "what comes next" part, and I actually found the directness refreshing.

One woman I met on Match ended up becoming a friend. She was from Maine, easy-going, outdoorsy, and sort of New Age. She taught me all about the healing power of crystals. Similar to my 4,000-footer quest, she was on a personal mission to hike the entire Maine portion of the Appalachian Trail in segments - about 300 miles in all. (What is it that draws so many of us to set out on these long outdoor quests?) We ended up seeing each other from time to time, mostly to go hiking. I think we each shared a similar voice inside our heads that this probably wasn't going to be "the one," but it was balanced, so that made things easier. She was very nice, and she baked excellent cookies...

So as winter transitioned to spring, the pain of my divorce was fading, I was enjoying the present (not just taking refuge in it), and looking to the future again. Somewhere along the line, grieving and emptiness had given way to rebuilding and hope.

A typo changes my life

If you're not familiar with online dating, here's a bit about how it works, at least on Match.com: First you create and post your own profile, and then you search around until you find someone else's that looks appealing. You can use all sorts of filters to narrow down your search criteria, such as age, interests, distance, and so on. I started out by entering a search distance close to home – say 10 or 15 miles. Not many prospects there – after all, it was mostly mountains and National Forest. So I kept widening my radius: 20 miles, 30 miles, 40 miles, etc. Well up there in the rural north country - how can I say this tactfully? – the pickings were slim, and I don't mean that literally. So I kept casting a wider net (sorry, that's a horrible image to use), until eventually I settled on a 100 mile radius. Yes, that's a long way to go to meet someone, but at least it got me into the more populated areas and small cities of northern New England. Even so, I started to see the same profiles over and over again, and not a lot of appealing ones.

One day I was doing a search, and all of a sudden my screen filled with a bevy of spectacular looking women. Wow! Where did all these beauties come from? I pinched myself to make sure I wasn't dreaming. Was this a gift from God, or was he messing with me? I looked more closely - many of the ladies had French sounding names. I checked my search radius, and found that I had inadvertently entered 200 miles instead of my usual 100. My typo had expanded my search to include the Montreal area.

Well the opportunity presented itself, so why not check it out? I started exploring. The women were indeed beautiful – for some reason the French-Canadian women look great, even in middle age. So much more chic and cosmopolitan than the ladies in rural northern New England. But as I read through their profiles, I started to notice a trend: Most seemed to fall into that same old pattern of just listing the things they like, all standard and generic. Despite their physical attractiveness, few of the women's profiles really grabbed me.

Then I noticed the pose. She was sitting in front of a big rock wall, wearing white shorts, with her knees pulled up and her arms wrapped around them. She had a certain gaze, sort of far off and dreamy, but with an engaging smile. (OK, in the spirit of full disclosure, she also had great legs.) I explored her profile. No corny clichés there - it was anything but generic. Now living in Montreal, previously in Europe, originally a prairie girl from Nebraska... interested in military history of all things... avid reader... sort of a quirky, witty humor... likes taking her bicycle on the train and hopping off at a great bike path - of course waiting until the train comes to a full and complete stop... I was intrigued.

We exchanged a few emails. Her name was Mary Ann. We got a good email conversation going, a light-hearted blend of curiosity, candor, and humor. After a while, I offered my phone number and invited her to call whenever she felt comfortable doing so. As she told me later, she had to get up her courage to make that first call. I never would have known.

First thing I noticed when I picked up the phone was her voice – unique, deep, didn't seem to fit her picture; to tell the truth, my first instinct was that she sounded older than she looked in her photo. Within a few seconds, however, I was enthralled in the conversation and forgot about her voice entirely. We chatted about our lives, how she ended up in Montreal, and where in the world Bretton Woods was. She told me about her career in international sales, and the extensive travel her job required. She started describing a high-stakes deal she'd been working on in India, then just like that she shifted into a pitch-perfect Indian accent: "I'm telling you, Sanji..." and so on. I just about fell off my stool. It was one of the goddamn funniest things I'd ever heard. Completely punctured any bit of pretense, seriousness, stiffness.

Instead of the usual restaurant setting for our first date, we decided to go for a bike ride. So one morning I loaded my bike onto the roof of my Subaru and drove up to Montreal - about a three hour ride. I had just parked and was taking my bike down off the rack, when I turned around and noticed this blonde woman standing there. Her head was tilted a bit to one side; she had a little half-smile - a blend of shyness and curiosity - and the most mesmerizing eyes I'd ever seen. Yes, time slowed down for the first second we met, and I still remember everything distinctly.

The rest was a delightful blur.

We rode along the bike trail next to the St. Lawrence River, chatting away at a leisurely pace. I noticed a little incline ahead, and told her I was going to sprint up it. "OK, you go right ahead, Lance." As I surged ahead, I chuckled to myself about the playful barb – I could tell already this wasn't going to be the same old thing.

Mary Ann showed me around Montreal, taking me first into the famous cathedral that hosted Rocket Richard's funeral and Celine Dionne's wedding. We popped into historic sights, markets, cafes, another church or two. She shifted back and forth between French and English without a hitch. I later learned she spoke five languages.

She invited me up to her condo, a funky loft in a charming old building overlooking the St. Lawrence River. Within a couple minutes, she somehow locked herself inside the bathroom, unable to get out. She pounded on the door, calling out about her predicament with a mix of panic, humor, and embarrassment - no doubt exacerbated by this being our first date! No sweat, I said. I found a little tool in her kitchen drawer, and calmly opened the lock – the whole thing took about thirty seconds. We laughed about the incident for the rest of our date, and still joke about it to this day. It was very revealing.

I visited her several times. We'd wander through her neighborhood in the old part of town – very quaint and European. We'd get take-out at a nearby gourmet deli whose proprietor we endearingly named "The Rude Guy." (That would become typical of us, assigning nick-names to the colorful cast of characters around us.) We sipped wine and watched movies, mostly documentaries on WWII. We had deep discussions about history and current events, increasingly mixed with playful banter. She asked about my teaching, and why I'd shifted from the academic to the business world. She talked about the high school teacher who introduced her to Thoreau, and how his writings opened up her mind and in a way, even her world. I helped her with some chores around the house such as fixing a chandelier, building a handrail for the steep stairway up to her loft, and of course replacing that finicky handle on her bathroom door.

Next trip up, I brought her a special gift from the little shop at Walden Pond: a book of Thoreau's political essays. She loved it. Home run!

On one of my early visits, Mary Ann asked if I wouldn't mind driving up to Quebec City with her. She'd purchased a kitten from a breeder up there, and she wanted to pick it up. "Sure, I'd be happy to go. Quebec's a beautiful city." Well, that's what came out of my mouth, but in my mind I was thinking, "*Oh no, I don't really like cats. Why couldn't it have been a puppy?*" When I saw the kitten, I could see why she'd already named him Gizmo. He was a tiny little Singaporean who looked right out of the movie Gremlins, with his huge ears and bug eyes. All the way back to Montreal, Gizmo drove us crazy meowing and crawling everywhere through the car, and climbing all over us, then settling into my lap, then curling up asleep, and by the time we got back to Montreal, I was smitten with the little guy.

A couple weeks later, Mary Ann made her first visit down to my place in New Hampshire. When she got out of her car, she asked my neighbor at the other end of the building which entrance was mine. Apparently, my ever-so-tactful neighbor told her to go around back because "that's the way the other women go." Oh shit! It's a wonder she didn't wheel around right there and drive back up to Montreal. When she came in, I noticed her eyeing a plate of home baked cookies on the kitchen counter. As I'd soon learn, she'd make a great investigator or spy – she doesn't miss a thing. Indeed, the cookies were from another Match date: The Maine Hiker. Oops!

Thankfully, we ended up having a great time. We talked and hiked and biked and explored my mountain world (so different from chic urban Montreal) and cooked and sipped wine on the deck and talked some more...

And when Mary Ann came back down for her next visit, you can just imagine the cookies she brought. Knowing her, she probably searched the entire world for the best cookie recipe. Yes, they were delicious! I won't tell you whose were better.

———◦———

What was that I said earlier about a "delightful blur"? Well that sure describes the next year and a half. It was a whirlwind. Visits back and forth across the border. Lots of work travel – mine around the US, Mary Ann's around the world. She got a second cat, a small Abyssinian she named Miss Peng after her tailor in Singapore. Between trips, her visits to Bretton Woods became longer. She stashed some clothes. I let my Match.com membership expire. I met her family. She met mine. My folks loved her. We hosted Thanksgiving. We hiked, skied, and hung out with neighbors. She set up an office in the spare bedroom. We brought in cubbies and stuff for the cats. And somewhere along the way - I can't remember exactly how or when, it was so seamless – she'd moved in.

Most of the condos up there were part-time ski places, many used primarily for rentals. Typical decor featured local wildlife scenes, retro ski posters, and often a pair of antique skis or snowshoes crisscrossed on the wall. Ours, however, was our full-time residence, so we started fixing it up accordingly. I built Mary Ann a walk-in closet, complete with ample storage for her impressive collection of shoes. I took apart the crappy condo-style wooden slat railing, and rebuilt it with stylish iron balusters and a milled oak handrail. That project took me months of painstakingly slow, meticulous labor – typical of me.

In total contrast, Mary Ann grabbed a bucket of paint and a ladder, and in 20 minutes painted over the moose and bear stencils from what she called "The Previous Regime." She got a kick out of that, and so did I. It was great to be able to chuckle about that without the slightest twinge of anything - that is, anything except joy for this new chapter of my life.

"Moving in together" soon evolved to much more than sharing a home. You move into a community as well. And Mary Ann did so, again ever so seamlessly. My neighbors embraced her, and she them. She met my ski instructor buddies, joining right in with the wise-cracking chatter. She volunteered as a Hospitality Host at the ski area - while I was up on the mountain giving ski lessons, she'd be unloading cars and greeting guests with her usual zest and flair. She met all sorts of people around our resort, and soon started introducing *me* to new folks – that was excellent!

I know the concept of "synergy" is an overused cliché these days, especially in the business world. But in our case, it really applied. Totally different in so many ways, we had one thing in common: Despite outward appearances, we were both introverts by nature. Somehow we played off each other, made a great team, and built a vibrant social network. Before long, we found ourselves at the center of things, deeply involved in the fabric of our community. Funny how up there in our remote little resort village, we ended up knowing far more people, and developing much deeper connections, than we ever did in the various cities we'd each lived in. I can't overstate how valuable that would become.

A bit more about our world up there: I've already mentioned the beautiful mountains and rivers and forests and sky, always a source of inspiration. Well the area was crawling with wildlife, too. Moose, bears, and foxes right out the window – sometimes even on our deck. The cats loved the constant wildlife show. Our little Miss Peng once went nose-to-nose with a 400 pound bear through the deck window – she fluffed and hissed and swiped her paw against the glass, and the bear backed away! One tough little cat.

In the midst of the natural wildness, the nearby Mount Washington Hotel was an oasis of culture and history. It was a majestic old place with a huge wraparound verandah and spectacular view of the Presidential Range. The grand lobby, with its bars and sitting areas, resembled the hotel in The Shining. It was a step back to a more elegant era – a place where you could meet visitors from around the world, get a good cocktail, and even dress up now and then. The hotel was famous as the site of the 1944 Bretton Woods Monetary Conference, where the Allies set up their post-WWII monetary and economic plans. I loved how Mary Ann was all over the history of the conference, reading, researching, and uncovering so many fascinating layers of significance. Typical.

Our local "big town" was Littleton – about 30 minutes away (if the roads were clear). That was the closest supermarket, drugstore, Home Depot, etc. Littleton had a quaint downtown Main Street with an old-time movie theater, a surprisingly good bookstore, and a sweet shop with the world's longest penny candy counter. It also had a nice little regional hospital.

Another important part of our world was the Manchester, NH airport - the gateway to our working lives. It was a bit under two hours' drive (again, if the roads were clear). We'd try to fly out of there if we could – Boston's Logan Airport was another hour further.

Mary Ann worked in the broadcasting industry. She sold audio processing equipment to radio stations and networks. Originally a TV and radio reporter, she'd transitioned to the sales side of the business and built an impressive career from there. Along with her unique voice, she had an exceptional ear for the nuances of sound. She developed a rare blend of technical knowledge, marketing savvy, and selling skills.

Hard-driving and high-energy, she charged headlong after sales with unrelenting passion. Creativity and personality, too.

Her forte was international sales. She knew how to navigate the complex world of international trade and customs regulations. Along with her language skills, she had a knack for understanding regional cultures and history. She traveled to an amazing array of destinations, not just the usual suspects like Europe and China, but more exotic places such as Madagascar, Sri Lanka, and Bangladesh. I could never grasp how Mary Ann managed to navigate her way around the globe so easily, yet at home she'd get lost on the local roads, or take the wrong hiking trail, or for that matter, get locked in her own bathroom! A baffling and endearing paradox.

My work travel wasn't nearly as exotic – usually just quick trips to your standard American cities for a couple days. After all those soul-less office buildings and airport terminals, it was always great to return to the uplifting scenery of our mountain world. But before long, I noticed something even more special about coming home: our comforting little rituals, our morning "coffee talks," our playful banter, the antics of our cats, and so on. Travel certainly does broaden your world, but it also makes you appreciate the simple things at home that you might otherwise take for granted.

One more thing I started appreciating: Mary Ann was a voracious reader, and she infused my world with ideas. Whether we were discussing history, politics, social trends, business, or just those silly lists you see on the Internet, we had amazing conversations. Sometimes they were like journeys, branching from idea to idea, exploring the deep connections between things. Other times they were quick, creative, filled with satirical humor and witty (or more often goofy) repartee. This brought a different kind of exercise to my mountain world. Yes, all the hiking and skiing was certainly making me fit, but it wasn't just my lungs and leg muscles that were getting stronger - I noticed that my mind was, too. Expanding, sharpening, stretching, enriching me into whole new realms.

Life can change in an instant.

Mary Ann and I were driving back from a long hike up and over North Twin, one of the 4,000-foot peaks on my list. We had spotted two cars at different trailheads, and she was following me home in her car. It had gotten dark. I glanced in the rear-view mirror to make sure she was behind me, then down at the speedometer. It read 52 MPH. Suddenly two dark shapes appeared out of nowhere in front of me – moose! No time to hit the brakes, all I could do was swerve – missed the first one, but *oh my god I'm plowing right in.* Funny how you hear the loud bang first, well before you feel the jolt, then a swirling tornado of debris, glass, entrails, screeching, flailing chaos. *So this is how it feels inside the last few seconds of life...* I heard a hideous wail. It was me. Then suddenly all was quiet. Deathly quiet. A few seconds passed. I took a breath and felt my chest move – only then did I realize I was alive. I pulled the handle and pushed against the crumpled door - it creaked open with a hard shove. I stumbled out and started walking back toward Mary Ann's car. For some reason I was holding my arms stiffly out from my sides, like a zombie. Then I realized why: I was covered in sticky blood, and I was holding my arms out so they wouldn't stick to my sides. I must have been quite a sight. Mary Ann stepped out of her car – I'd never seen her so speechless.

Other cars pulled over. Someone called 911. I sat on the guard rail. I had little twinges of pain, but I thought I was OK overall. The EMT's arrived. They looked me over and suggested I go to the Emergency Room to check for deep cuts and internal damage. I said sure, that made sense. I gave Mary Ann cursory directions to the Littleton Hospital – she'd never been there before. The EMT's strapped me into the ambulance. Two stocky middle-aged ladies with cigarette smoke on their breath and gruff, north-country accents, they used salty language and kept calling me "hon" (as in short for "honey"). They were excellent.

A state cop popped his head into the ambulance – said I'd hit an 800 pound female, and she was dead. I felt sad for the moose, and even sadder for her bereaved companion. The cop asked me if I wanted the meat. "Huh?"

"That's how we handle moose kills – the driver's entitled to the meat."

"No thanks, you can have it." As the ambulance pulled away, I chuckled to myself about the wonderfully quirky world we lived in way up there in the north country.

From the first moment the hospital staff wheeled me into the ER, I got the sense they'd done this many times before. They had such an orderly process, with everyone knowing exactly what to do. Their teamwork was reassuring. So was their calm and pleasant manner - so unlike the dramatics you see on all those TV hospital shows. They explained what they were doing each step of the way. They took my clothes somewhere to shake out the glass, then put them in the wash. Wearing little jeweler-like eyepieces, the doc and his team went over me inch by inch, pulling out pieces of glass with tweezers. He said all my cuts were superficial – no stitches needed. Then, to make sure they got out all the tiny shards, they ran a small vacuum cleaner over my body. It tickled! We all had a chuckle over it. Then they sent me to take a shower, after which they bandaged the larger cuts. As they finished patching me up, someone brought in my clothes, freshly washed and still warm from the dryer. I joked that it felt like a luxury spa. The staff got a kick out of that.

As I was getting dressed, they brought Mary Ann in from the waiting room. I still remember the look of trepidation in her eyes, immediately softening with relief when she saw I was OK. Then, when I told her how they vacuumed me, she burst into her radiant smile, and we both started laughing. We've laughed about it ever since. As a matter of fact, if you ever get a chance to meet Mary Ann, ask her about my moose collision – I bet the first thing she'll mention is the vacuuming part!

That was the first of many health scares and challenges we faced together. It taught us a lot: To remember the fragility of life, and how everything can change in an instant. To appreciate the great first responders and healthcare folks who go about their jobs with such competence. To realize the power of humor. And of course, on the more pragmatic side, to drive carefully at night on those dark mountain roads!

I don't think I've told anyone this, even Mary Ann: I was fortunate to have survived the collision. The car's air bag didn't deploy because the moose's tall spindly legs offered hardly any resistance to the sensors in the grill. The entire impact was its body plowing into the windshield at 52 MPH, shattering the glass and buckling back the frame. The ER staff said they'd seen many fatalities from moose collisions exactly like mine. Not to get gruesome, but they explained that the typical cause of death is the moose's body pushing through the windshield frame and breaking the driver's neck. In my case, my eyeglasses were shattered and my nose was cut, but the impact stopped right there. They said another few inches would have had a much worse outcome. I'm glad I had a Subaru – one tough vehicle.

You really start wondering when you have a close call like that. Why did I survive? Was it something more than the strength of that windshield frame? I'm not a prayerful person in any conventional type of way, but I do feel gratitude to some sort of spirit. And I sure felt it that night. Gratitude to have survived. Gratitude that I wasn't out there alone on that dark road, or in a long taxi ride back from the hospital to an empty house. Gratitude to have Mary Ann in my life. And strange as it sounds, even gratitude that we went through that frightening experience together - somehow it deepened our bond.

As Mary Ann drove home (ever so slowly) from the hospital, we didn't talk all that much. In great part that was because we were both gazing wide-eyed out the windshield, scanning for dark shapes in the road. But I was also quietly reflecting on life's amazing twists, not only how I'd survived such a close call that night, but how I'd been granted the gift of a makeover in life. How this spectacular woman from Nebraska by way of Europe and Montreal had somehow found her way to my remote little world in the New Hampshire mountains, and into the Emergency Room by my side, and now here we were, driving through the dark night back to the warm comforts of our home, to the promise of tomorrow, building a life and a future together.

And to think it all started with a typo.

Yes, life sure can change in an instant. In so many ways.

Reclaiming Mt. Willey

It was a gray Saturday morning. We were a little groggy - we'd been at a party the night before and had a few drinks. (And I know what you're thinking - yes, I drove home *very* carefully!) It was mid-December in what had so far been a mild winter. (Winter begins around late November up there.) Despite what I said earlier about my 4,000-footer quest being a slow journey, I was getting itchy to finish the list before full winter conditions set in. I had only one peak left: good old Mt. Willey. The weather wasn't great that morning, but at least there wasn't much snow. I mustered my best motivational skills to pull Mary Ann away from her coffee and paper and get her to climb it with me: "How 'bout it, sweets? What do you say we give it a shot? This could be my last chance to finish the 4,000-footers before spring. You know how much climbing Mt. Willey means to me – and I'd really like you to be up there with me when I do it." OK, I admit I was flagrantly "playing the Mt. Willey card," and all that that meant. At least that was my cover story.

Mary Ann grumbled a bit, but she agreed to come along. Soon we were trudging up the muddy trail. As we gained elevation, the mud turned to slush, then to icy crust, then to solid blue ice covered by a few inches of snow – the most treacherous footing of all. I stopped to put on my crampons. Mary Ann kept moving, relentless as always. The trail got steeper and steeper - soon it was almost like a frozen waterfall. I called up to remind her to get those crampons on. She kept inching upward, too scared to stop. I was starting to think of what I could do to catch her in case of a slip. Finally she found a little ledge where she put on her crampons, and we scampered up from there.

We could barely tell when we reached the top. It was heavily forested, covered in a foot of crusty snow, shrouded in thick fog, with total visibility maybe 50 feet. All that marked the summit was a rock pile and a rustic wooden sign. We had a quick little celebration. I took out my list of the 48 peaks and snapped a photo. As I focused the camera, I noticed my fingers were shaking. It wasn't that big a deal to complete the list of the 48 peaks, at least the physical accomplishment – many New England hikers do that. But in my case, the symbolism was meaningful, and I felt a little surge of something inside.

A small rock jutted out from the crusty snow. We huddled there and wolfed down a sandwich. Now that we'd stopped climbing, the cold was setting in – a damp, raw type of cold that chilled you to the bone. I could tell Mary Ann was getting antsy to get moving again. I walked over to my backpack and fumbled around for the little box. Finally I found it, and brought it over to the rock where she sat. I knelt down in the snow in front of her, and took out the jade ring from Singapore that my mother had given me. I don't remember my exact words - I'm sure they were a shivering jumble anyway - but I asked Mary Ann to marry me. Her eyes flew wide open, she exploded into her spectacular smile, and she blurted out "Yes!" We had a few hugs, snapped a photo or two, and then in unison I think we both said, "OK, let's get the hell off this miserable mountaintop!"

Despite the treacherous footing, we seemed to float down the trail. By the time we got halfway down, it was pitch dark. Fortunately, I had packed headlamps. Also fortunately, I had pre-loaded the fireplace awaiting us at home...

———

The snow finally came that winter. And by late June, as we stood on the back verandah of the Mt. Washington Hotel, there were still patches lingering on the Presidential Range above. It was a small, intimate ceremony, with close family members and a few friends – 20 people in all. Low key. Not at all conventional. The Justice of the Peace was a sweet 80-year-old lady from a little town nearby. Mary Ann's dress came from a shop at the Singapore airport. A ski instructor friend played acoustic guitar. No photographer – just a few guests snapping pictures. We did have a couple nods to tradition, such as a candle lighting ceremony that got our nieces and nephews involved - we thought that was nice. We also had a cake-cutting ceremony, although our cake was unusual. It was shaped like a ski hill, and the bride and groom figurines were little plastic skiers! Yes, a bit unconventional and goofy – sort of like us.

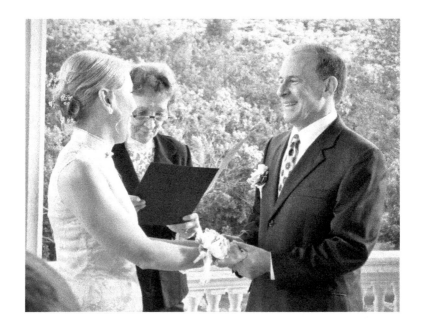

I guess it's not standard wedding protocol for the groom to give the wedding toast. But my two brothers and I had already gone through one rotation of being best man at each other's wedding, and now we were in uncharted territory with this being my second. Hey, I was 53 years old, and there was a lot I wanted to say about my bride, so I said what the hell - I'm going to give the toast myself.

As you might guess by plowing through this book so far, my toast was on the long side. I got lots of heckling from my brothers about it. (That's one of the nicest things about my family. We make fun of each other - in a good-natured way.) I kept a copy of my words that afternoon, and they still resonate perfectly, maybe even more so, now many years later. I'll spare you from having to read the whole toast, but here are few excepts that I think capture the essence of Mary Ann, and summarize what she meant, and still means, to me:

> *...To a woman who negotiates million-dollar deals in far-off lands without flinching, yet at home her heart melts when she sees a lump under the bedspread with a little paw sticking out...*

...A woman who, for all her worldliness and brilliance, doesn't take herself too seriously, and occasionally reveals glimpses of that shy, scrawny bookworm who was always picked last when choosing up teams in gym class...

...And finally, a woman who has proven to me that it's never too late, and you're never too old, to laugh with abandon, to believe in miracles, and to be reborn.

A fateful transition

It's hard to describe exactly, but something was different after that ceremony at the Mt. Washington Hotel. Different and better. Sort of a lessening of uncertainty, a more solid foundation underneath, more confidence toward the future.

Between work, travel, and our busy lives, we never had time to take a real honeymoon vacation that first year. But that didn't matter, for two reasons: First, we could step right out our door into a resort paradise, a destination that attracted people from all over the world, often for their own honeymoons! Why travel when we were already here?

Second, our whole marriage seemed like one big honeymoon so far.

Even so, there was one thing gnawing away below the surface: Mary Ann's work was going stale. After many years of high-flying success, she had recently gone through the wringer of organizational politics and management changes, and now found herself in an environment that lacked stimulation. Some people are fine working in a maintenance type role, being a caretaker of the status quo. She's not. She's motivated by (and gifted at) driving growth, developing markets, innovating new products, creating buzz, creating period. But now she was losing the passion, and the work and international travel were becoming increasingly draining.

At the same time, big changes were afoot with our resort. New owners had recently bought the whole place. Their vision was the complete transformation of our remote little valley into a world-class resort destination. They brought in a real estate development group from the South to build a village, condos, and homes. Their plans and renderings were spectacular. One of the top hotel executives knew us pretty well, and he kept suggesting that Mary Ann consider joining their real estate sales team. He felt that she would be a great spokesperson for their vision, living the resort lifestyle right there on site, able to connect with the high-end clientele they were looking to attract.

We held that option in our back pocket, debating the pros and cons. Meanwhile, Mary Ann kept working and traveling.

Then two game-changing incidents happened.

Mary Ann had dual US/Canada citizenship, with a passport from each nation. She'd typically choose whichever passport made things easiest with border control and customs in each country she visited. In those days, she frequently used her Canadian passport, because the US invasion of Iraq had soured our relations with many nations around the world. Late one night she arrived at the airport in Sri Lanka, radio equipment and her Canadian passport in hand. Suddenly the customs agents whisked her away into a little room, where they proceeded to interrogate her. The questioning got harsh - several agents pointed automatic rifles at her just a few inches from her head!

What was going on? Well, there was a separatist rebel group in Sri Lanka called the Tamil Tigers, much of whose funding and support came from Canada. The agents accused Mary Ann of smuggling communications equipment to them. For once, she'd chosen the wrong passport.

After several hours, she finally convinced them she wasn't a rebel sympathizer, and they let her go. They pretty much tossed her out on the sidewalk in front of the airport at 3:00 am, not a taxi or anyone in sight, except for a few creepy guys going back and forth eyeing her.

How's that for a "road warrior" travel story? Makes flight delays and crowded airplane seats seem like small potatoes, doesn't it?

PS – She still ended up making several good sales on that trip. I told you she's relentless.

Mary Ann's next international trip took her to a remote region in China up near the Mongolian border. A day or two after she returned to Bretton Woods, she started complaining of an earache. I brushed it off as jet lag, and gave it the typical "take some aspirin, get some rest" response. I went back to whatever I was doing, and didn't think much more about it.

When Mary Ann woke up the next morning, she said her earache was really bad. She wondered if she should go to the doctor. I was scheduled to ski instruct that day, and I wanted to go over to check for my lessons. I was expecting a private request. (These are special lessons where a guest had specifically asked for me. Not only was the pay higher, but they were a sign of good client relations and professional accomplishment. I had built up lots of them by then, which was a source of quiet pride.) Mary Ann said her pain was so bad she didn't feel well enough to drive herself to the doctor. "OK, OK, just let me run over there and take care of my lesson. Then I'll come right home and we'll see how you feel." I headed over to the ski area in my typically dutiful manner, arriving right on schedule, as always.

When I came back home a couple hours later, Mary Ann was still in bed, which was very unusual for her. Her earache was worse than ever, and she looked horrible. "Let's call your doctor and see if we can get an appointment today."

"No, this feels real bad – I think we'd better go straight to the hospital."

"OK. Let me get out of these ski clothes and take a quick shower, and we'll go." Just then, she rolled over, and I saw her pillow was soaked in blood. Holy shit! I jumped, and we were out the door in seconds – I was still wearing my ski clothes.

Once again, I noticed the competence of the ER staff. They wheeled Mary Ann right in, started an IV immediately, hooked her up to the monitors, drew some blood and sent it off to the lab. They kept things moving briskly, but always maintained a calm manner. I also noticed one thing they didn't do: They gave none of those empty reassuring phrases like "You're gonna be fine." Instead, they talked in concrete terms about what they were doing, and what would come next. That impressed me.

The ear specialist doctor soon came in with the lab results. He

43

looked concerned. He told us that Mary Ann had a severe infection in her inner ear, and there was an alarming wrinkle: They were unable to identify the particular strain of bacteria – he speculated that it might even be unknown to Western medicine! He said he'd get her started on an intravenous antibiotic, but it was just his best guess if it would work.

As they started the IV drip, I glanced over at Mary Ann. She was hooked up to all sorts of tubes and wires. She looked exhausted and pale, but still managed a weak smile and a wise-crack or two with the staff. Seeing her like that touched my heart - I actually said a quiet little prayer to myself...

After an anxious hour or two, it appeared that the antibiotic was working. The ear doc came back in, and only then told us the full story. He said it was the worst ear infection he'd ever seen. It had spread almost all the way through her inner ear, and was headed for her brain. He estimated that she had about another 10-12 hours left – after that, it would have most likely been fatal.

Wow, another close call. That made me stop and reflect. I was horrified by my lackadaisical response to her earache complaints, by the way I kept plodding along at my own pace, stuck in my little routine – by the way it took a bloody pillow to jolt me into action. There's an art to listening, *really* listening, like with a capital "L" - and this was a perfect example of my *not* doing so. To think the consequences almost killed my wife. That was an eye-opener.

Well, the one-two punch of the Sri Lanka interrogation and the ear infection scare were the last straws. Mary Ann soon made the decision to leave her job and start working with our resort's real estate group.

It was a tough decision for her. She wasn't just letting go of a job and a career, but also a source of her identity and self-esteem. As in any major transition, she faced a period of uncertainty, anxiety, even self-doubt.

At the same time, the promise of her new job was huge. It gave her the potential to make good money, plus the satisfaction of selling something she believed in passionately: the resort paradise right outside our door. She dove right in with her typical energy, studying like crazy for her real estate exam (she even made 3x5 flash cards), and acing it on her first try.

Like so many things in life, you don't always realize the full significance at the time. But in hindsight, OMG, did Mary Ann's career change turn out to be a fateful move, in so many ways. First, I had been on her health insurance plan at her previous company, and thanks to the COBRA law, I'd be able to stay on it for 18 more months. Second, the community connections we'd already built up would help greatly in her new job, and she'd continue to expand that network; that would turn out to be valuable in ways far beyond selling real estate. And third, most important of all, she'd be home.

The springtime of promise

So there we were in the spring of 2008. Life was filled with promise.

Mary Ann had stepped off her career trajectory to take a chance on an exciting new real estate venture, one that would allow her to stay closer to home, be with her new husband, and hopefully make good money. A new career where she could combine her marketing and sales brilliance with her knowledge of our local area. She was reinvigorated.

Always networking for potential leads, she'd extended herself even more deeply into our community. She volunteered to give Historical Tours at the hotel, she continued to be a Hospitality Host at the ski area, and she joined the local women's Book Club. Everything was in place for her to thrive.

My corporate training schedule was booked almost solid for the rest of the year, with workshops and clients lined up all over the place. I always liked having a lot of work booked ahead of time. That provided some financial security, and also allowed me to interweave my work travel with my busy schedule at home, including community service, social events, and of course ski instructing.

Speaking of ski instructing, with a few seasons under my belt now, I'd become an "old pro." I'd built up lots of regular clients, and I was enjoying the camaraderie, fun, and satisfaction more than ever. Even my skiing had gotten half-decent for a creaky-kneed middle-ager. I'd just finished up a great ski season, celebrating the final day with my instructor buddies over at Wildcat.

Having completed my 4,000-footer hiking quest, I was set to take my mountain exploits to a whole new level. That fall I was signed up for an expedition to the Kangshung side of Mt. Everest, a remote wild face of Everest that had only been climbed twice. We had no intention of venturing anywhere near the summit, but we were planning to ascend to 21,000 feet, getting views of the world's highest peak from a rare vantage point. Seeing Mt. Everest was one of my life-long dreams.

On the national backdrop, young Barack Obama was bursting on the scene with his "Hope and Change" optimism. The economy and stock market were still chugging along, Bear Stearns and Fannie Mae to most eyes just little blips under the radar.

Mary Ann and I were in our ninth month of marriage, still newlyweds in every way, still in that delightful dream-like state where it hadn't fully sunk in that we were actually married.

The pain of losing my first marriage and being displaced to the mountains was now not only a distant memory - it seemed like another life. I'd healed and rebuilt, better and stronger than ever. My mother had certainly been right with her Thanksgiving guarantee a few years before – I'd found happiness I never dreamed of, and then some.

Life was filled with promise in the spring of 2008.

I went in one morning for my annual physical exam, almost swaggering with confidence awaiting the usual affirmation of my health and vigor. And then the doctor's office called me back the next day to take that second blood test.

Our world was about to unravel...

Part 3

UPHEAVAL

Getting the news

So that brings us back to my meeting with Dr. Diener, in early May of 2008, to find out the results of my bone marrow biopsy. In particular, why had my blood counts veered off course?

I waited in the exam room, sitting on one of those exam tables covered with a roll of crinkly paper. Dr. Diener popped his head in the door. "We'll come back here later to do the exam, but why don't you come down to my office first." He walked me down the hall into his office, then closed the door behind us. He gestured for me to have a seat in front of his desk – the chair was soft and comfortable. Nearby were several photos of him and his wife – I noticed they liked to do active outdoor things together. I asked him about that. It was more than the standard chit-chat you have in any meeting before you get down to business. Something inside was telling me that it might be helpful to ask a little about *him*, to connect at a more human level - maybe the discussion we were about to have would be hard for him, too.

When our chit-chat reached a natural pause, I had a pretty good idea of what was about to come. Diener took a breath, and in a calm, gentle voice he said, "Well the test results are back from the lab, and

I'm afraid that you have cancer." I wasn't surprised – Mary Ann and I had spent the previous week researching the Internet and doing our homework. All the signals were there. Even so, hearing the words "You have cancer" was a jolt. *Me, cancer? Mr. Outdoors - the picture of fitness and health? How could that be?* That denial lasted all of a second or two. It took about another two seconds to realize, and accept, that life was about to change – big time.

In some crazy way, part of my reaction was relief – at least the uncertainty of the past few weeks was over, and now we had something tangible to work with. The "C" word was finally out there in the open. Beyond the initial jolt, I don't recall feeling any particular emotion at first - in typical fashion, my mind was already racing ahead, driven by pragmatism, craving more information.

Dr. Diener was right there with me. He explained that, in clinical terms, I had something called Myelodysplastic Syndrome. Before I could get out the words "What the heck is that?," Diener started translating it into human terms, again in his calm, kindly manner. My mind was swirling and I had a hard time focusing, but I heard something about abnormal blood counts and white blood cells and defective things called blasts, all very possibly developing into leukemia. Leukemia! Well that struck a nerve. My mind shot back 45 years to the first time I ever heard the word "leukemia," to the shock of hearing on the Channel 5 evening sports report that one of my boyhood football idols, Ernie Davis, had suddenly died from it. The childhood terror that had been embedded deep within for all those years suddenly erupted, and I felt a shiver of fear. My mind raced ahead again. "So what does this mean? What's my outlook?"

I remember Dr. Diener's words distinctly: "Well, you're going to need a bone marrow transplant." What he didn't say in words, but tacked on with his body language and intonation and everything else, was the additional phrase, "...in order to survive." I heard it loud and clear.

My immediate reply was, "So where can I get one of those? Can you do it?" In my typical manner, the "where" came before the "what." I had no idea what a bone marrow transplant was, but I was already leaping ahead to the next steps. I've found the question "Where do we go next?" to be a powerful way of coping with (or skipping past?) the emotion.

Dr. Diener referred me to... well, I probably shouldn't say where, but it was a highly respected hospital, probably the most logical choice in the area. He said he'd heard that they'd recently brought in a "rising star" new doctor to head up their transplant program. "Should I call them to make the appointment?" I asked.

"No, let my assistant handle it," he replied. "That'll get you in sooner."

Diener took me back into the exam room. He gave me a once-over, saying I looked strong and healthy - at least on the outside. I told him that I felt a little off lately, with increasing fatigue and shortness of breath. He referred me to take an EKG stress test to make sure my heart and cardio system were OK, and ready to handle the rigors ahead.

As I left Dr. Diener's office, I thanked him for being so kind and direct in handling my initial diagnosis. I wondered if I'd ever be back.

That night I made the call to Mary Ann. She was on a trip down South with her real estate colleagues, looking at various resort developments that would be the model for ours. With all her anxiety over her new job (not to mention being a thousand miles away), you can imagine how she felt hearing the news. I tried to share my own look-on-the-positive-side perspective: "At least the uncertainty is over, and now we know what we're dealing with." Well, I'm not sure that helped her leap past the emotion the way it does with me – we're not exactly alike in that regard.

The next week was something like an extended version of my moose collision - a swirling jumble of calls to family members, Internet searches, books and websites to check out, information coming at us from all directions. Amidst all the confusion, we learned the basics about bone marrow transplants: They'd need to find me a matching donor, I'd have a long hospital stay, the treatment would be rough, the recovery would be long, and the chances of survival far from certain.

I couldn't wait to get into the hands of the hospital to learn about the details and, most importantly, take the next steps.

During that week of jumble, I went back to the Littleton Hospital for my stress test. They hooked me up to all sorts of electrodes and wires and monitors. I kidded that I felt like one of those astronauts in the early NASA days. They asked me to start striding on a machine that was like a combination treadmill and stair stepper. "Just keep going as long as you can. We'll keep raising the level until you tell us to stop. And remember, the machine always wins."

As I started stepping, I occupied myself by trying to make sense of all the beeping sounds and numbers and graph lines flashing on the monitors. The technicians kept raising the speed and incline. I kept going. The beeping got faster and faster. They cautioned me that they were going to bring the machine to its highest level. I kept on striding. Finally they turned it off. "Well, Peter, you made history. You're the first person ever to beat the machine!" I laughed it off with some light-hearted wise crack, but on the inside I was doing a quiet celebratory fist pump.

I'm not telling you this to be boastful (well, maybe just a little), but rather for two other reasons: First, to show how all that outdoor exercise had made such a difference - I was still in pretty good shape, even with my recent deterioration. That would give me a big advantage making it through the physical challenges to come. Secondly, there's also a lesson in there about the importance of goals and benchmarks, and celebrating (quietly) your accomplishments, even the little ones, in the midst of a long struggle. That stress test was a major milestone, something I looked back on as a source of motivation during my eventual recovery. On the flip side, it also ended up being a pinnacle of sorts, a bar so high that it's been unattainable ever since.

A tale of two hospitals

The day finally arrived. We made a point of getting there way ahead of time. We'd done enough research about the transplant process to know that I'd be spending at least a few weeks in the hospital, maybe a month or more. So before going to the hospital itself, we wanted to check out the area where Mary Ann would be staying when she came to visit me. Her environment would be as important as mine. Come to think of it, actually more important.

We found a nice Courtyard hotel where she could use our substantial pile of Marriott points. Nearby was a grocery co-op, which had all sorts of interesting local produce and cheese and meat – all the stuff we could rarely get way up where we lived. I even joked that this almost made the whole transplant worth it. Mary Ann slapped me down for that. (Even with her great sense of humor, she's always been the enforcer of sensible boundaries for my jokes.) There were a few half-decent looking restaurants within walking distance. Also a bookstore, very valuable for her. Beautiful mountain vistas. It all looked great. I was relieved.

When we saw the sign for the hospital entrance, I felt a little shiver and took a deep breath. We turned in, and immediately noticed the beautiful landscaping - it was like driving through a park. The signage was colorful and easy to follow. The hospital lobby was spacious and filled with light. There was a coffee shop with tables out front, like a sidewalk cafe. A guy was playing piano. As we made our way down the hall to the check-in area, we noticed huge colorful tapestries on the wall. There were large picture windows with views of distant mountains. We'd heard a lot about what a great hospital this was, and we were starting to see why.

We registered at the check-in desk, then they directed us to another counter where they took my insurance information. Someone walked us to the exam room. As we sat waiting, several staff members came in with various forms for us to fill out. A few times they asked us to complete the same form we'd just filled out earlier. Someone else came in asking if I brought my medical records and labs - there was some confusion locating them. No, I'd sent them in several days ago, and called to verify they'd arrived. *Hmmm...*

Finally the doctor came in. I noticed that his greeting wasn't particularly engaging – no eye contact, barely a hand shake. He started talking about bone marrow transplants in very general terms. Most of what he was telling us wasn't new – we'd already done our Internet homework. I was waiting for him to focus on my own situation. But he kept going on, almost like he was giving a lecture and we were faceless students way at the back of the lecture hall. He asked us no questions, and didn't acknowledge the particulars of my case. We kept listening patiently, passively.

After a while, he stepped out, saying that the insurance person wanted to talk with us. She came in and asked us many of the same questions we'd already answered at the check-in area. She stepped out for a few minutes, then came back in with more questions and forms. Mary Ann asked her something about whether the treatment would be covered. "It depends on your insurance," was the reply. I caught Mary Ann's eye – she was not amused.

The doctor came back in. "*OK, now he's going to get down to the nitty gritty,*" I thought. But the lecture continued, as wandering and aloof as ever. I started tuning out. Here we were, meeting the doctor who would lead the team to save my life, and I actually found my mind drifting off, if you can believe that. Eventually we (vaguely) got the sense he was getting ready to wrap it up, and I finally mustered up a question: "So where do things stand with my case? What's the next step?"

"Well, let's see where things are in about six months," he replied. "We'll get back in touch with you then to schedule another appointment. And by the way, if you don't hear anything from our end, give us a call to remind us." As we made our way out to the car, I don't think we even noticed the beautiful mountain views.

On the ride home, we discussed how something just didn't feel right with the whole visit. I was concerned about the lack of specifics. Mary Ann said how violated she felt when the insurance person came into the exam room. As a typical guy, I was oblivious to it at the time, but I could see how she felt: There she was, discussing (ostensibly) the treatment to save her husband's life, and into the same room they march in someone to discuss insurance. Not the most tactful way to handle it.

And what about the "call back in six months" part? That seemed like an awfully long time to wait, especially considering what Dr. Diener said about the severity of my condition. We wondered if the doctor didn't want to take my case for some reason. Maybe he thought he couldn't save me. Maybe our insurance didn't check out and they were trying to steer us away. Or maybe they just didn't know what they were doing. Who knows? The mind fills in the blanks.

The thing is, we were still assuming this was where we'd go for my treatment. It was *the* place - the mecca for all things medical in the area. Thank God we ended up listening to our gut instincts nagging away inside. And thank God for Walter.

Walter was a fellow ski instructor. He lived outside Boston and came up every weekend to his cottage near the ski area. He'd been an instructor at Bretton Woods for years, in fact decades. Walter knew everybody. He had the gift of gab - a warm laugh, a twinkle in his eye, a classic Boston accent, and a heart of gold. A retired school principal, he had a certain way of commanding attention and taking charge.

We told him about our hospital visit and our gut feeling that something wasn't right there. I'll never forget Walter's words: "Pedah, get yaself to Dana Fahbah. Get yaself to Dana Fahbah." Translated into normal (i.e., non-Boston accent) English, that meant, "Peter, get yourself to Dana Farber." He was referring to Dana Farber Cancer Institute in Boston. I was certainly familiar with it, mostly as the home of the Jimmy Fund, a long-time New England charity that raised money for kids with cancer. Anyone growing up in New England knew all about the Jimmy Fund – the Red Sox had been one of their main supporters for years. All those photos of Sox players visiting with bald-headed kids in the hospital really touched your heart.

Anyway, I knew Dana Farber was a renowned cancer center, but it was way down in Boston, three hours away. Walter wouldn't let up: "Pedah, there's only one place to go. Ya gutta get yaself to Dana Fahbah." He's a persuasive guy. So we said why not - let's check it out. What else were we going to do? We had six months to fill.

Mary Ann made some calls and got us an appointment within a

week or so. The morning arrived. We fueled up our plastic to-go mugs with high-test coffee, and made the long trek down to Boston. From the outskirts of the city on in, we crawled through thick morning traffic. Dana Farber Cancer Institute (DFCI) is located in a medical area densely packed with hospitals, narrow streets, congested traffic, rude drivers, and pedestrians scurrying everywhere. We slowly made our way through the maze and into the parking garage, where we had to keep circling down and down deep below ground to find a space. We ended up being late for our appointment. The lobby was crowded and confusing. We had no idea where to check in. The first person we encountered was a young lady sitting at an information desk, chewing gum, head down, immersed in a gossip magazine. When I asked her for directions, she barely looked up as she gave us a disinterested point down the hall. *Hmmm...*

We finally found the check-in desk. They had everything prepared as if they were expecting us. Well that was reassuring. They took my insurance card, entered some information, and gave it back within thirty seconds. (The topic of insurance never came up again.) The receptionist confirmed the details of my appointment, then asked me to hold out my wrist. She snapped a hospital wrist band onto it. Wow, that was a jolt of reality!

The waiting area was a crowded madhouse, with hospital staff scurrying to and fro, and many patients standing against the walls. We squeezed into a couple seats. We started looking around. I noticed many of the patients were wearing masks, some looked gaunt, many were bald or wore head scarves. What a diverse group: a mix of all ages and ethnicities and body sizes and shapes and social-economic levels and styles of dress. One thing almost everyone had in common, however, was someone by their side. I squeezed Mary Ann's hand.

We started talking to a guy wearing a Yankees hat. He had a gruff, classic New York accent – not at all like the Boston accent. He said he came up here for his treatments. That told me a lot about DFCI. We both joked about his venturing into the heart of "enemy territory" wearing the logo of the dreaded Yankees. He said everyone was warm and welcoming – his Yankees regalia always led to some good-natured chatter in the waiting room, just like now. We started talking about baseball, the rivalry between the Sox and Yankees, and how we saw the rest of the season going. They called him for his appointment. As he got up to leave, we shook hands and wished each other good luck – we left it unspecified whether we were referring to the baseball season or other things.

They called us into the exam room. The team got right to work checking my vitals and verifying my information. The intake doctor who'd been assigned to my case came in with my labs and the biopsy results from Littleton Hospital in hand. (I'll give him the pseudonym Dr. Intake.) No lectures. He gave me a quick once over, poking and prodding here and there, and asked me to do a few simple physical tasks. Then he reviewed my chart. I could tell he was concerned. He said he wanted to do a second bone marrow biopsy to compare the results to the one from Dr. Diener, which was now a few weeks old. The trend between the two would help determine the next steps. That sounded impressively sensible to me. Still in the mindset of first hospital's pace, I asked, "So when would you like me to come back down for my biopsy?"

"No, no, no. We're going to do it right now. Unhitch your pants and go lie down on that exam table over there."

They booted Mary Ann out of the exam room. No, "booted" sounds too harsh – they were more tactful than that. No matter - she would have left on her own; she has a hard enough time with regular IV sticks – watching that tool drill into my backside would have been too much. Anyway, as I lay down on the table, I noticed the biopsy tools already laid out neatly; the nurse immediately started prepping the entry spot, the doctor stood by at the ready, and I thought to myself, *"This is the place I want to do my transplant!"*

The bone marrow biopsy was no big deal this time – I was already getting used to the procedure. (I would end up having two more.) We made an appointment to come back down in a week to get the results and discuss the next steps. This was starting to feel familiar.

As we drove home, we reflected on the two hospitals. "What were we thinking," we asked ourselves about the first place. "A rambling lecture from the lead doctor? Discussing insurance in the exam room? Making us wait six more months? Asking us to call back to remind them? You've got to be kidding!" The contrast with Dana Farber was startling, and our decision was a no-brainer. The rush hour traffic was horrible as we crawled our way out of Boston and onto the long road back up to the mountains. But that didn't matter – we knew we were in good hands. And we knew we were going to have to get used to making that drive many times.

After we got home, Mary Ann and I did some additional Internet research. We found that the first hospital had done a total of eight bone marrow transplants – Dana Farber had done over 1,500!

That led us to all sorts of realizations about handling health challenges - call them "lessons" if you'd like: Do your homework. Seek out and accept suggestions and references. Beware of first impressions, especially the superficial stuff. Trust your gut instincts. Speak up. Ask questions. Don't just ride along passively – take charge of your care. After all, when you look for a new refrigerator, you read Consumer Reports and on-line reviews, check out models at Lowes, ask the salespeople questions, etc. Why not take the same type of approach with your cancer provider?

And a few words to anyone who works in a cancer hospital: Have an organized system for taking in new patients. Be prepared. Be decisive. Communicate clearly. Train your doctors to engage with patients and their caregivers, to empathize with how they feel and what they want to know. And sure as hell don't talk about insurance in the treatment room!

Maybe most important of all, minimize uncertainty. Provide tangible, concrete information. Uncertainty is like a Petri dish, a fertile breeding ground for anxiety, stress, and fear. In my opinion, uncertainty can be just as damaging as the cancer itself, maybe even more so.

For what it's worth, the first hospital not only lost us as a patient, but they lost a ton of revenue.

Reshuffling the deck

It was another anxious week as we waited for our next trip down to Dana Farber. A week of more Internet searches, calls, cards, and spreading news. Amidst all that, good old Walter did something else that ended up being very special. He introduced us to one of our condo neighbors named Tommy, a fellow we'd never met. (As I said before, Walter knew *everybody*.) Tommy had had a bone marrow transplant several years before. He couldn't have been any warmer or more gracious. He started calling from time to time, just to check in. He never told us what to do or how to feel – he just answered our questions when we asked, and always radiated good cheer. That was so valuable, connecting with a real live person who'd been through a similar experience. Talk about alleviating uncertainty.

The week finally went by, and Mary Ann and I drove back down to Dana Farber to learn the results of the biopsy. Dr. Intake came out into the crowded waiting room to find us. He walked us to a quiet area. He looked deeply troubled. It seemed he was having a hard time getting out the words. I actually found myself comforting him: "It's OK doc, you can just tell it to us straight." He said the biopsy findings were alarming – the trend between the two indicated rapid deterioration in my blood readings. The cancer was getting real bad real fast. I didn't think to ask whether it had transitioned from myelodysplasia to leukemia. No matter the name of the condition - it required urgent action. He said we needed to get moving immediately on the search for a bone marrow donor. In fact, behind the scenes, the DFCI folks had already gotten everything ready to start the search – they just needed my approval to set things in motion. "Hell, yes! Where do I sign?"

Meanwhile, he said he was going to start me on chemotherapy immediately, cautioning us that this was "palliative" at best. I didn't know what that word meant, but it seemed to make sense given the context. The goal was to slow down the progression of my cancer to buy them time to locate a matching donor for my transplant. That could take weeks, months, or... never.

Dr. Intake explained how the chemo infusions would work: Four or five days a week, several hours each day, a week on, then a week off, repeating for at least a couple months. I was amazed how much time they'd take up. Yup, my life was sure about to change. He gave me a choice where to get the chemotherapy. I could come down to their infusion suite in Boston, or he could send the chemo order up to my local hospital in Littleton. Easy decision – I chose Littleton. So I'd be going back to good old Dr. Diener and his oncology clinic after all!

On the ride back up to New Hampshire, Mary Ann and I reflected again on the first hospital. We were more stunned than ever to think they were going to wait six months before even seeing me again – from what we'd just learned, that probably would have been a death sentence. Whew, that was scary. We talked about schedules and the changing logistics of our life, especially now that I'd be spending so much time at the chemo clinic. That kind of pragmatic talk always kept *me* focused.

What I don't think we talked about enough, I now realize, was how Mary Ann was really feeling on the inside. I can only imagine. She'd uprooted her life in Montreal, moved to the mountains, gotten married for the first time, taken on a whole new career, and, less than a year into her marriage, now this. In hindsight, I guess I wasn't the only one with frightening stuff churning deep inside.

Anyway, we kept chatting away as we made our way northward on I-93. Suddenly I saw blue lights flashing in the rear-view mirror. I pulled over and rolled down the window. A NH state trooper ambled up – a burly, square-jawed, tough-looking officer right out of central casting. He asked if I knew I was going 83 MPH. (The speed limit was 65). "No, officer, I'm afraid I was a bit distracted." I held my arm up to the window. "See that band on my wrist? Well we just spent the day at the hospital down in Boston, and we learned that I have a long cancer fight ahead. I guess I was a little preoccupied, and I just wanted to get home." I glanced up at the officer. His eyes were welling with tears. He started telling us about his sister's battle with cancer. A tear rolled down his cheek. We chatted for a while, cars whizzing past. We wished each other good luck, and he sent us on our way.

By the way, my response to the officer really was spontaneous and sincere – that's exactly why I wasn't paying attention to my speed. Of course, as I drove away (at a steady 63 MPH), Mary Ann and I started wringing the humor out of the incident. "Wow, you really played the cancer card there," she kidded.

"Yes, pretty well, I must say," I replied. We still chuckle about it to this day. In fact, I still wear my hospital wrist bands on the drives home from DFCI, where I continue to go for my regular check-ups. The running joke is that I can use it to talk my way out of a speeding ticket. Of course, I'd never really do that. Actually, I wear my wrist bands for quite a different reason: as a private little reminder to appreciate the gift of life I've been granted. In any case, we haven't been stopped again since.

We soon got a letter from Dr. Intake to his patients, saying that he had decided to leave direct patient care and return to his previous field of cancer research. Seeing how hard it appeared for him to break the news to us, we speculated that maybe he just wasn't cut out for the interpersonal parts of cancer care. After all, I'm sure there were plenty of patents with news a lot worse than mine. His letter assured us that our case would be handed over to the appropriate staff at DFCI. We awaited the next steps, and turned our attention to reshuffling the cards of our life.

It was a tough call to make. I had always found mountains inspiring. The Rockies, Sierras, Alps, even the good old Whites right out our window – mountains always stirred my soul. Laying eyes on Mt. Everest had been a lifelong dream. Much more than just another bucket list item to check off, this had been almost like a spiritual pilgrimage for me. The trekking company was great about refunding my deposit. I thought of that Langston Hughes poem about a "dream deferred." I hoped "deferred" would turn out to be the right word.

An even more difficult call was to cancel my work gigs for the rest of the year. I kept one on the books for the open week between my first two chemo rounds, but after that... Well, it was best to wipe the slate clean to be prepared for whatever may come. It was hard to cut the cords of stability, and drift off into the unknown. It was also hard letting go of the income. Mary Ann's real estate venture was still in its early phase, and much of her pay would be based on commissions. More uncertainty there. Also, we were starting to hear rumblings in the housing and financial markets, though we had no idea of the extent to which the bottom was about to fall out from under the economy.

Speaking of Mary Ann's work, of course she wanted to give her employers a heads-up on my health situation. When she told the CEO of her development company, he said all the right things – concerned, compassionate, and reassuring. The executive who recruited her was equally gracious and supportive. Her direct supervisor at the sales office, by contrast, suggested that she resign. One more harbinger of challenges to come...

The morning of my first chemotherapy treatment, I packed up a little knapsack with my laptop and a book. Mary Ann headed out for her work at the real estate office, sharply dressed as usual in a resort-sporty way. As we walked out together, suddenly we both started chuckling. For the first time ever, we were like a conventional couple heading off to our respective jobs for the day. In typical fashion, we played up the humor. I made some crack about my stylish "briefcase." She encouraged me to "Have a good day at the office, dear." We laughed, gave each other a little kiss, and headed off our separate ways. Come to think of it, all the humor aside, in a way this actually *was* my new job.

Once again, I received a warm welcome at the Littleton oncology clinic. Somehow it felt good to be back. When the nurse walked me into the infusion suite, she introduced me to all the regulars there as "the newbie." I got a kick out of that. The suite had lots of windows and about five or six infusion chairs. I settled into mine. It was an adjustable recliner, very comfortable, like a high-tech Lazy Boy. There was a TV above, and a little holder on the arm for the clicker. Next to the chair was an infusion pole with all sorts of tubes, hooks for IV bags, and a beeping monitor. Outside the window, the flowers were in full bloom.

The nurse started an IV in my arm. Then she brought in the plastic bag of my chemo and connected it to one of the tubes on the pole. She went through a series of checks and double checks. I'd heard horror stories about the ravages of chemotherapy, the way it messes up your stomach and all that. As the nurse started the IV drip, I braced myself for stinging or nausea or something. But I didn't feel anything. I was surprisingly comfortable relaxing in that chair on my first day of palliative chemotherapy, reading, channel surfing, gazing out the window at the early summer flowers, wondering what lay ahead. It was June 30th, 2008 - our first wedding anniversary.

The summer of anxiety

Thus began our summer of anxiety.

We knew Dana Farber was working on the donor search, but we didn't hear anything from them for a while. We waited as patiently as we could, trying to fill the void of uncertainty by staying occupied with our daily lives. Mary Ann immersed herself in her real estate work with her usual energy. Though the developers didn't have anything tangible to sell yet, she was making contacts, generating leads, creating buzz around the exciting changes to come. That helped keep both of us focused.

I led my last workshop, a two-day business writing program down in Massachusetts. Though I was starting to feel fatigued, I'm sure nobody noticed. Actually, it turned out to be a surprisingly refreshing "escape." More difficult was sending out that final invoice and closing out my books for the year.

We finally heard from Dana Farber that they planned a meeting in a couple weeks for us to meet our entire transplant team. That was exciting! What a relief to have something tangible to look forward to – sort of an antidote to the uncertainty. They asked for my brothers' contact information so they could bring them in for marrow donor testing. Siblings generally provide the best chance for a good donor match because of the genetic similarities. This was another encouraging step forward. We waited anxiously to hear the results.

Mary Ann and I continued to enjoy our outdoor activities together, though I could feel myself slowing way down. My red blood counts were declining rapidly - these are the cells that carry oxygen throughout the body. I assumed this was the cause of my increasing fatigue. I noticed that the walk up the hill to our townhouse was getting harder, and before long I had to take rest stops along the way.

As the summer progressed, we received a huge outpouring of support from friends and neighbors. This took many forms: phone calls, cards, emails, CD's and DVD's, drop-by visits, offers to do errands, and all sorts of other great gestures. Lots of advice, too: Call this person, read this book, check out this website, eat this food, take this supplement, do this type of meditation, join this church... All the accumulating advice became a bit overwhelming, but we tried to appreciate that it came in the spirit of good intentions. At least most of it.

First meeting with the transplant team

I'll always remember the letter we got from DFCI confirming our meeting with the transplant team. The tone was warm and welcoming. It listed the people we'd meet, their roles, topics we'd discuss, the types of questions we might want to prepare, etc. That gave us a clear roadmap of what to expect – certainly an anxiety reducer for a couple venturing into the unknown of a potentially scary meeting like this. That letter gave us confidence, not only toward the upcoming visit itself, but in the whole place.

We learned that the doctor who would be leading my transplant was Robert Soiffer. Unlike our first visit to the other hospital, this time we wanted to go in prepared, so we did a little homework. We learned that Dr. Soiffer was the Chief of Hematologic Malignancies, or something like that. That's a fancy way of saying he was the top blood cancer guy. He was also head of some national associations, as well as a professor at Harvard Medical School. (DFCI is a Harvard teaching hospital.) Impressive background, obviously knew what he was doing - we were in good hands. At the same time, a little voice inside my head was wondering why did we get such a top-level doc? Could that have been a signal about the severity of my case? As I said earlier, the mind tends to fill in uncertainty with all sorts of dark thoughts.

Well, the second he walked in, any anxiety we might have had dissolved away. Dr. Soiffer was completely down-to-earth, warm and engaging. He explained things in a calm, simple manner. He asked us questions, and took the time to answer ours. He seemed competent and confident enough to let a little personality show through – totally professional, but human. There's an art to that. (On the ride back home, Mary Ann would point out how she loved his colorful tie and rumpled shirt – so humanizing and endearing.)

Dr. Soiffer updated us on the donor search so far. Both my brothers had been tested by this time, and he gave us the disappointing news that neither turned out to be a match for me. In an ironic twist, however, they ended up being a perfect match for each other! We all exchanged a few wise-cracks about that, though inside it was quite a letdown. (I think my brothers were even more disappointed than me. They so much wanted to do something to help, and now that option was taken away.)

Soiffer explained Plan B: If siblings don't match, next they search among donors with the same racial and ethnic ancestry. This typically gives the best chances of finding a good match, due to similarities in genetics and blood proteins and other complex things that I don't understand. Their testing had pinpointed my ancestry to be Ashkenazi Jewish. (I had never known about the first part of that phrase until I learned about it at this meeting.) They were currently searching for a match among registered donors of that background. It's interesting how this is one area in which ethnicity really does matter.

Though he never made us feel rushed, I knew Dr. Soiffer had other patients to see. A few times he stepped out gracefully, while other members of the team would step in and talk with us. The whole process flowed smoothly – impressive teamwork. It was helpful to meet the different providers who would be involved in my treatment – each offered valuable information and suggestions. Unlike the first hospital, however, nobody mentioned insurance.

One of the head nurses came in and gave us a huge binder. It made a thud when she put it down. The binder was jam packed with information about every aspect of the bone marrow transplant process. At first glance it looked overwhelming, even intimidating; but the nurse immediately put us at ease by focusing us on just the most important parts. She particularly emphasized the period *after* I'd return home from the hospital, especially the critical first hundred days. Due to my weakened immune system, I'd be quarantined in partial isolation; it would be essential to keep everything clean and germ free; my diet would be severely restricted; and so on. There was a lot for us to know and do - especially Mary Ann. But the way the nurse guided us through that binder really helped - it was more like a pleasant conversation than a lecture. As a result (months later), we ended up remembering everything!

While we were chatting with the nurse, suddenly Dr. Soiffer popped his head back into the exam room. "Come on out here, Peter. I'd like you to meet someone." I stepped out into the hall. There stood a frail looking woman, all bundled up in a mask and scarf and gloves – almost like a mummy. At first I wasn't even sure if I could talk directly to her. Soiffer introduced us and said she'd had her transplant 30 days ago! I was stunned. We started chatting. Even though her voice was weak, she exuded warmth, zest, life. Said she felt great. Can you imagine the impact that had on me? I'll never forget it.

Dr. Soiffer soon returned to the exam room. He and the nurse continued to answer all our questions, with no rush. Finally, as we were about to wrap up, I took a deep breath, mustered up a bit of courage, and asked him to walk us through the mortality figures. I made sure to call them "the statistics" rather than "my chances." There's a big distinction there.

First, he estimated the likelihood of finding a donor match for me was about 65%, based on the number of registered donors out there with my Ashkenazi heritage and a few other factors. (We didn't discuss what the options were for that other 35%, though it certainly crossed my mind.) Assuming I got a donor, the statistics indicated I'd most likely survive the hospital stay for the transplant, though it was by no means certain; I remember having a fleeting thought about not making it out of the hospital. Then Soiffer explained that the next two years would be the most critical period, to the point where the survival rate was about 50%. The statistics for making it to the five-year mark dropped a bit further, though I don't remember the exact figures. I do recall, however, running through the numbers in my head, thinking about the obvious – you can certainly imagine.

I'm sure Dr. Soiffer noticed me mulling over the numbers. As we headed out, he leaned over, gave me a little tap on the shoulder, and said, "You'll do great." For some reason, I believed him. And I mean believe with a capital "B." It was like when my mother gave me those encouraging words at Thanksgiving a few years before. Somehow you just know.

Mary Ann and I headed home, confident in the team, the place, and the plan. Everything was set. All we could do now was go about our lives as best we could, and wait...

The cookout

One day we walked over to a big summer cookout at the ski area. The ski slopes were covered in wildflowers. The sweet smells of grilled burgers and hot dogs filled the air. Many of the winter staff had returned for the party, having swapped ski wear for flip-flops and t-shirts. Everyone had a beer in hand.

Right away I started sensing sideward glances, eyes darting away, something a little off with the vibe. You can just feel it. One of my ski friends – a warm, always-jovial woman – soon came running over and gave me a big hug. "Peter! It's so great to see you! So how are you doing?" That's not always an easy question to answer when you've got cancer. I summarized my prognosis as directly as I could, with the bottom line that I was doing fine. She looked surprised. Then she explained why. The word on the street was that my cancer was terminal and I had only a few months to live. Wow - no wonder everyone looked so uncomfortable seeing me!

I asked her to spread the word that I had every intention of returning to the slopes, maybe not that upcoming winter, but certainly the next one. I promised we'd take a run together.

That was quite a wake-up call about the power of rumors. It was like a real-life version of that telephone game we used to play as kids, where a phrase changes as it passes from person to person - one more reminder of how misinformation tends to take root amidst uncertainty. So I decided to do a better job of letting everyone hear the true story directly from me. A friend suggested I start a blog. I had no idea how to do that – I'd always thought of bloggers as people inhabiting a different world. But I soon found a blog site and figured out how to use it. Later that day, my first post was online.

That blog would become another one of those action steps I took that ended up making a huge difference. And I'd like to take you there in a moment.

So the next part of this book, its middle section, is more of an "in-the-moment" narrative. I'll let my blog posts (and some photos) tell the story. Almost everything is exactly as I wrote it at the time. I've changed some names, chopped out some extraneous stuff, and made a few minor tweaks so a general reader will understand what I'm talking about. But otherwise, this is how I saw events unfolding in real time. I thought you might get a kick out of experiencing the heart of the story this way – sort of like the POV style they use in filmmaking.

Now I didn't always realize the significance of things at the time, and some important things I left out altogether. So from time to time, especially at the major transition points, I'll jump back in and add a few observations from the perspective of present day hindsight. I'll also summarize and condense certain sections, just to keep the story moving along.

The original name of my blog was Peter's Cancer Journey. Not a very imaginative title, but as I look back on it, that word "journey" certainly turned out to be appropriate. Don't expect a crisp, linear story, but rather a meandering odyssey with all sorts of side roads. You'll also notice several premature attempts to bring the blog to a close. Much like "false summits" in mountain climbing, there were several places I thought I was ready to wrap it up, only to find the story kept going. I guess there's a lesson in there about the difficulty of finding closure in cancer journeys, at least those like mine. So brace yourself for some false summits.

So let's go back to late July, 2008, amidst our summer of anxiety.

Mary Ann was trying her best to stay focused on her new real estate job. I was spending lots of time at my chemo treatments. Our transplant team at Dana Farber was in place, and the donor search was going full tilt. Everyone was waiting. The rumors were swirling. The phone kept ringing. It was time to start letting the world know how I was doing. So here we go back to my original blog posts. Enjoy the journey.

July 29, 2008 – Welcome!

Hello, and welcome to my first post.

Well the last few months have been quite a ride. A ride where your life unexpectedly veers off course and you're not sure where you're going to end up.

It all started in April with a routine physical exam in which my blood test results were "a little off." From there I bounced from one test and to another, first trying to pin down the cause of my low blood readings, then coming to accept the reality that I have cancer, and now facing the prospect that I could be in a heap of trouble.

Fortunately, I've found my way into the hands of some great cancer specialists down at Dana Farber in Boston, and they're taking aggressive action. Most important of all, I've got Mary Ann by my side - she's a rock. As anxiety-filled as this ride has been, I have to say we're doing OK so far.

Anyway, I decided to start this blog for several reasons. Mostly just to keep everyone updated, and to get at least some sense of staying in touch when I can't respond to every email or card right away. Also to answer your questions, to clear up some false rumors I've heard, and even to keep some sort of a chronicle about this journey we're starting.

A couple weeks ago I barely knew what a blog was, let alone how to create one. But thanks to a friend's advice, here I am. So I'll give it my best shot. I'll keep adding updates from time, so come back and visit often. Feel free to leave a comment or question under any of the posts.

Thanks again for visiting. Here we go.

July 30 – What exactly is my disease?

I've heard a lot of rumors out there about my condition, so let me try to give some factual information. In the simplest terms, I have a form of blood cancer. Something has gone wrong in my bone marrow (the place where blood is produced), and as a result I'm experiencing increasing abnormalities and deficiencies in my blood cells. My initial diagnosis was something called Myelodysplastic Syndrome. Sounds pretty obscure, eh? What this means is that my red cells, white cells, and platelet levels are not reproducing normally, and I have an increasing number of defective cells called blasts appearing in my blood.

This condition is sometimes a precursor to leukemia. As a matter of fact, my blood numbers have been deteriorating so rapidly that I think I may now have something called Acute Myeloid Leukemia. I haven't gotten the exact diagnosis lately, but the name of the disease really doesn't matter at this point. Without a successful bone marrow transplant - which I'll describe in an upcoming post - my outlook is not good.

But contrary to some of the rumors going around, my cancer is *not* terminal! Bone marrow transplants do often work to cure my type of disease, and I hope to get one soon. They just need to find me a matching donor. The search is underway, and we're waiting anxiously.

In the meantime, I'm taking some preliminary chemo to slow the advance of the cancer. I'm still able to function pretty much normally, though I've been feeling weaker and more fatigued lately.

August 3 - Please consider registering to be a bone marrow donor

One of the most inspiring things about this whole adventure has been the willingness of countless friends and neighbors to offer your bone marrow for donation, and even organize donor registration drives in your communities. I can't begin to describe how deeply this has touched Mary Ann and me. While the chances that your particular marrow will be a match for *me* are miniscule, registering to become a donor is still a great thing to do to help others in general.

Here's why: The doctors told us that I have about a 65% chance of finding a matching donor, based on my ethnic heritage, the number of potential donors already registered, and various other factors. Many other blood cancer patients, especially minorities, have much lower chances. So the more potential donors in the "pool," the greater the chances for all of us so afflicted to find a match.

Let me explain a bit about how the process works. First, you get your tissue tested using a procedure called HLA (human leukocyte antigen) typing. The procedure is simple. You get a little kit to swab your inner cheek with Q-Tip like things, you stick on some bar code labels, and you send it to the lab in a pre-paid envelope. Easy! They record your readings in a huge registry. You can then remain registered as a potential donor as long as you'd like, or withdraw at any time. If your tissue type ends up matching a person in need, they do some further tests, and then they harvest stem cells from your blood or marrow to transplant into the patient. The harvesting process is no big deal – usually it's just like an extended version of donating blood.

For much more information about the whole testing and donation process, check out the National Marrow Donor Program's website at bonemarrow.org, and also the Gift of Life program at giftoflife.org. And please spread the word to as many people as possible.

August 5 - How a bone marrow transplant works

Pretty much the only hope I have to survive this disease is to get a bone marrow transplant. And for that to work, they need to find a donor whose marrow is a suitable match for mine. (See the previous post on bone marrow donation.)

The Dana Farber Cancer Institute currently has a team searching the world's donor registries for a match for me. If they find one, they'll make arrangements to harvest stem cells from that person's marrow or blood, and then send it to Boston.

In the meantime, I'll go through various preliminary tests and procedures, then check into the Dana Farber transplant ward for approximately a month-long stay. I call this my "spa vacation!"

During the first part of my stay, I'll receive extremely heavy doses of chemotherapy for a few days, followed by several more days of total body radiation. The goal of these procedures is to kill my current blood cells. Apparently I won't feel so great during this time.

Once my cells are killed off, the transplant team will infuse the donor's stem cells into me intravenously. The new cells will somehow make their way into my bone marrow, where they'll hopefully start reproducing properly. The whole process is sort of like getting an oil change for your car - flush out the old, replace with the new.

The period after the transplant itself is the most critical part. If the cells reproduce normally, my blood readings will start returning to healthy levels, and within a few weeks I'll regain my strength enough to go home. This doesn't always happen – sometimes the new cells just don't take.

Sometimes various side effects and other diseases arise. And some patients experience Graft vs. Host Disease, which is like an internal rejection battle between the old and new cells. In extreme cases, this can be fatal.

During my hospital stay, my immune system will be severely hindered due to my lowered white blood cell levels. I'll be extremely vulnerable to germs and infection, so I'll be confined to a sealed-off transplant ward with limited physical contact with the outside world. Should be interesting.

Anyway, the doctors have been refreshingly blunt about risks and mortality statistics - not everybody makes it through the transplant process and its immediate aftermath. At the same time, they've also been very encouraging that my overall fitness and health put the odds in my favor that I'll survive. I guess all that hiking and mountain exercise has helped!

Now, they just gotta find me a donor...

August 6 – Life while the donor search goes on

Life continues for Mary Ann and me as normally as we can make it under the circumstances. She's loving her work with the resort real estate group. Can't beat the commute to the office (two minutes!), and she's thrilled about all the exciting plans for our resort. She's plunging into it with her typical energy – probably a good thing to keep her focused on something besides my disease. It'll also be a good thing for their sales once their plans turn into something tangible – she's an amazing salesperson, in her own special Mary Ann type of way.

No more work or travel for me, so I'm spending lots of time at home puttering with woodworking projects and trying to be a good "house husband." Although I get tired and winded more than usual, I'm still able to do moderate activity – with plenty of rest breaks.

August 14 - More chemo; still waiting for that donor somewhere

Nothing new on the search for a donor. We're trying to keep the anxiety under control - the best way is to go on living as normally as possible. Lots of tennis playing lately. Mary Ann has been taking lessons and is really improving, especially on the forehand side. I huff and puff a lot while shuffling around the court these days – glad her shots are getting more accurate!

I've been spending lots of time getting chemotherapy infusions at Littleton Hospital. These aren't intended to cure my cancer, but just slow down its progression to buy time to find a donor. Aside from fatigue and an upset stomach, no major problems – even my hair is still there! It's been surprisingly pleasant going to my appointments each morning. In the photo you might be able to see that I'm reading a book on the Marx Brothers. Mary Ann and I love their zany humor and scathing satire – especially therapeutic these days. The folks at the Littleton Hospital have been great - they give me complete control of the clicker so I can switch between all the Olympic sports on TV. I'd like to take that reclining chair home one of these days!

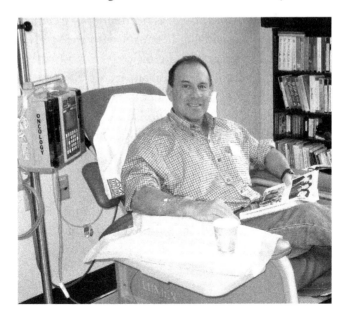

August 21 - A false scare

Today Mary Ann had a rare day off, so we decided to go for a bike ride. Because of my condition, we have to choose our ride routes carefully. I'm feeling a lot weaker lately. My red blood cells are low, which means I'm not able to process oxygen normally, and I get out of breath very easily. I cannot do long, hard climbs anymore. (Sorry, "anymore" sounds too final - I mean "for the time being.") So we chose the Presidential Rail Trail in Gorham, which follows an old railroad bed below the northern Presidentials. Very smooth, gentle grades, etc. Should be no problem.

About a mile into our ride, I was lagging way behind, feeling far more fatigued than expected on such level terrain. Something just felt wrong, and I started getting concerned – even a bit scared. This was all happening so fast. I finally caught up to Mary Ann, who was waiting for me at a road crossing. I could tell she was discouraged by how much I was struggling (though she would try never to show it). I started to ride ahead so she wouldn't see the tears in my eyes.

Soon I had to stop again for another rest. Really discouraged - hard to believe I was already this weak. As I bent over panting for breath, I noticed that my front wheel was on crooked, and it was rubbing against the disc brake. No wonder I was having such a hard time! So I straightened out the wheel, started rolling smoothly down the trail, and we ended up having a nice ride through the beautiful terrain below Mt. Madison and Mt. Jefferson. Whew!

Anyway, I'm still plugging away these days, trying to keep the anxiety and hopes and fears in check, savoring the time I spend with Mary Ann, living life, doing what I can, accepting what I cannot.

Sept. 1 - A special family visit

September now begins up here with the most beautiful weather imaginable. There's a little hint of fall in the air, and the hillsides are starting to become dotted with red foliage. With the month changing, I realize it's been quite a while since my last entry. I guess I've been waiting to get more definitive news before writing again, and to tell the truth, we haven't heard much lately - the donor search and waiting continue, along with the anxiety.

But that's OK, because yesterday I had the type of day that made me feel good to be alive, and I'll write about it instead. My brother Larry drove up for the day from Concord, MA with his family and our parents. That's about a 350 mile round trip with six people in the minivan, all to spend a little time with me. First we just hung around the house watching videos from the kids' summer camp. Then we pulled Mary Ann away from her work to join us for lunch at the golf clubhouse – the hot dogs were awesome, and we sat a table away from local ski hero Bode Miller.

The highlight of the afternoon was a hike along a secluded stretch of the Ammonoosuc River, where the water has carved deep pools into the granite. The sun was warm, the water was crystal clear, and it didn't take much prodding for Lily and Sam (our niece and nephew) to plunge in. Although the initial shock of the icy mountain water appeared to be quite a jolt, they soon got used to it. They're both strong swimmers. I enjoyed watching them exploring the river's nooks and crannies, struggling against the swirling currents, floating down the natural smooth granite waterslides, and leaping (carefully) off the rock ledges into the deep pools below.

If I were feeling my normal self, I would've jumped in there with them. But now, it was great just to sit on the ledge and watch. My parents sat on the rocks a bit further back from the river's edge, smiling peacefully. There was something magical about sharing that river gorge with three generations of family members, watching the young ones frolicking in the water below with such playful abandon, all of us just living so purely in the moment.

Sept. 10 - America at its best

Still nothing to report on the donor search, so let me switch to a more uplifting topic. One of the most gratifying things about this whole experience has been the willingness of others to help in any way they can. That response has continued to grow, as countless friends and even people we don't know have told us they've gotten tested, registered as donors, etc.

We've been amazed how people of so many different backgrounds have taken the initiative to spread awareness of bone marrow registration through their various networks. Just a few examples: My sister-in-law Marcia contacted a regional director of rabbis, who then wrote an eloquent plea to all the rabbis under him, who in turn will spread the word to their congregations during the upcoming Jewish holidays. My ski instructor buddy Billy has started a prayer chain through the Catholic church that's apparently spread across the country. Mary Ann's sisters have contacted work colleagues, various Catholic organizations, and alumni networks. My long-time grade school chum Johnny G tapped into his contact list of old schoolmates, and as a result, I've heard from people I haven't seen since the third grade! One of my clients, Nationwide Insurance, has initiated a bone marrow drive among their thousands of employees, and they've even linked up with a similar effort sponsored by NASCAR.

It's so uplifting to see how this effort has unified so many diverse people under a common purpose - to help others. To me, this is America at its best.

Now if you'll please allow me a little editorial comment. Ever since the Republican convention, I've been watching VP candidate Sarah Palin going around repeating the same snarky speech in which she implies that anybody different from her is not a "real" American, and she dismisses "community organizing" with a sarcastic sneer. Well, Palin's divisive politicking aside, it seems to me that all you folks who've been spreading the word about bone marrow donation among so many diverse groups actually embody the best of what community organizing, and the *real* America, are all about! Thanks for your efforts!

Sept. 12 - They've found a donor!

Today has been one of those days when you feel the earth shift.

I received a call this morning from the search coordinator at Dana Farber. She asked me if I was sitting down, then broke the news that they had identified a "perfect match" for me! I can't begin to describe all the emotions that swept through me. I'm usually a laid-back guy, but as soon as I hung up the phone I became a blubbering basket case - jumping up, punching the air, screaming, laughing, crying. I guess a lot of that anxiety that's been bottled up all summer came spilling out.

I called Mary Ann at work, who for one of the few times I can ever remember was stunned speechless. Can you believe it? Mary Ann was speechless! Well at least for a few seconds. Then she screamed, and apparently threw something across the office, scoring a direct hit on her startled colleague. Then she came running home.

We canceled our plans to go to a dinner party tonight, and instead decided to order in the greasiest pizza we can find, watch a Marx Brothers movie, drink a few beers, and not clean up anything afterward.

As for the donor, they keep the whole process confidential. All we know is he's a 22 year old male, which makes *both* of us happy, if you know what I mean.

Two huge caveats: First, the donor still has to be willing to go through with the donation process (occasionally they back out), and second, he has to pass a physical and undergo some preliminary treatments. The search coordinator said it's very unlikely these will be problems, but the whole thing is not yet chiseled in stone. That's OK - I'd much rather have the uplifting news of things suddenly moving ahead (even if we get let down) than continue with this summer's awful anxiety of waiting and wondering.

For all of you who contributed to this wonderful moment, whether through marrow testing, gestures of support, prayers, funny cards, quiet good wishes, "community organizing," or however else, our eternal thanks.

Sept. 20 – A bonus from borrowed blood

Well it's been a little over a week since we got the thrilling news about the donor match. Nothing new to report - we're still waiting to hear if the donor passes his physical and consents to move forward with the donation. I'm confident he will, but there's always that nagging little anxiety in the back of your mind.

Meanwhile, this past week was filled with another round of chemotherapy - back in that comfortable reclining chair every day. I also got a "bonus treatment" today. My red blood count has recently dropped to dangerously low levels, making me feel extremely sluggish and out of breath. I've barely been able to walk up the little hill on the road to our condo – I have to pause for breath about every five steps. So they had to give me a blood transfusion in addition to the chemo - almost eight hours in that chair! The goal was to infuse some borrowed blood into me to boost my red blood count, if only temporarily.

When the nurse started the transfusion, at first it felt strange seeing that bag of someone else's blood dripping down the IV tube into my arm and my own bloodstream. But I noticed no ill effects, and soon felt a bit better with all those extra red blood cells carrying oxygen through my system - sort of a legal form of blood doping, I guess.

This evening I took a walk with Mary Ann, and I immediately found myself huffing and puffing a lot less than usual. We walked across the street to the ski area and started hiking up the gentle beginner slope. I felt OK, so we continued on. Soon we were at the base of Darby's Drop, a steep expert run. "Let's give it a shot," I said, so we kept trudging upward, right up the steep pitch. It was amazing how good I felt – almost like old times. When we got to the top, Mary Ann and I stood there silently, holding hands, savoring the sunset glow. She said my face looked less pale. So my thanks to the person who so generously donated that blood, even if it only provided a temporary illusion of feeling better. I hope I'll be able to hike back up there again someday with my own red blood cells.

We expect to get a call this week from Dana Farber saying that things are moving forward, and hopefully giving us a date to begin the transplant process. My best guess (or maybe I should say *hope*) is that I'll be going into the hospital in mid-October. Of course, I'll keep you posted.

One more thing that I hope keeps moving ahead: Just because it looks like I've gotten *my* match, please don't stop spreading the word about donor registration. Think of all the thousands of other people who are going through the excruciating anxiety that Mary Ann and I did the last few months. You'll be helping them out by spreading awareness and expanding the pool of potential donors. Thanks – keep it going!

Sept. 30 - **Still riding the roller coaster**

In my last entry, I said something about that "nagging little anxiety" we were feeling while waiting for the next bit of news. Well ten more days have now passed, we still haven't heard anything more, and that anxiety isn't so little or nagging anymore. This has been a real roller coaster ride, from the thrilling high point of hearing about the donor a few weeks ago - to sliding back down into another period of waiting and wondering, and yes, even worrying.

As that Tom Petty song says, the waiting is the hardest part. Frankly, it's probably been toughest on Mary Ann. It doesn't help that she's now the sole breadwinner in a new job in a new career in an emerging organization selling high-end second-home resort real estate in these troubled financial times - can you imagine the stress? I've been amazed (and proud) that she's been able to function at all.

I've probably had the easier of it. I fill my time with medical appointments and puttering around the house working on various projects. For example, I've been slowly building a little entertainment cabinet out of locally grown maple and cherry. I have no idea what I'm doing, so I tinker away at my own pace, figuring it out a little bit at a time - very calming and therapeutic.

Another way I've recently occupied myself is to play accountant. I've plunged into our mounting pile of insurance claims, medical bills, and expense records, trying to get a handle on it all. This might help us at tax time. It also feels good to have some sort of purpose.

In the process, I've come up with some interesting statistics about this whole adventure. Since I first got an inkling I might be sick back in April, I've now made 34 separate trips to doctor's offices or hospitals. We've driven a total of 2,200 miles for these trips. Our total medical bills have surpassed $100,000 so far. Just a week of chemotherapy costs about $17,000!

Fortunately, we have good medical insurance, which so far seems to be covering most (though far from all) of the costs. During this period, that insurance has cost us $2,400 in premiums. We've already had to pay about double that amount out-of-pocket for co-pays and non-covered expenses. And I'm sure all these costs are a drop in the bucket compared to what's coming once I go in for the transplant.

Back to the furniture building project.

Oct. 5 – Finally, a (tentative) hospital admission date!

While we were going through all the anxiety I wrote about in the last post, the wheels were still turning behind the scenes at Dana Farber. We assumed that they were, but it sure would have helped if they just let us know every now and then. Reminds me of a good bit of wisdom my father used to say about running his small business: Even if you don't have anything new to report to your client, it's still good to check in with them every now and then just to give a little reassurance. It's incredible how the void of not hearing anything allows so much worry and anxiety to take hold.

Anyway, for the first time Dana Farber has given us an admission date, if still tentative at this point: They told me to be ready to go on Friday, Oct. 24. Wow - how exciting! A bit scary, too.

Meanwhile, two nights ago Mary Ann treated me to a birthday dinner at the nearby Mt. Washington Hotel. It's a fancy place, and we got all dressed up. As we were getting ready for them to bring the check (so I thought), the lights suddenly dimmed, the wait staff approached our table with a birthday cake, and the whole place started singing "Happy Birthday." Usually I feel this is sort of hokey, but not this time. I was deeply touched, especially because I believe the staff knew all about my situation (another example of the great community spirit where we live). After I blew out the candles, I saw tears in Mary Ann's eyes. She leaned across the table and, her voice quivering, asked, "We'll be back here to celebrate your birthday next year, right?" All I could manage to stammer out was "absolutely."

Oct. 10 - Hospital admission draws nearer

For all you blog visitors who are not fortunate enough to experience the spectacular fall show in northern New England, I wish you could see this. The colors, especially the reds, are incredible this year.

The seasons up here never cease to amaze me. A few entries ago, I used the phrase "in the moment." Well lately, in the midst of all the wondering about the future, I've found myself stopping to savor all the beautiful natural scenery around here more than ever. I guess it's pretty obvious why.

Anyway, I've gotten two more bits of news:

First, the Dana Farber folks called and scheduled an Orientation Day for us on the 15th. This will be a full day of medical tests, labs, a tour, and meetings with the transplant doctor and various oncologists and nurses and social worker. Sounds impressive and exciting – hopefully not too overwhelming. Mary Ann kidded that it'll be like going to Freshman Orientation all over again!

The other news is that the insurance company called today - they confirmed that my treatment has been determined to be a "medical necessity." When I heard that, at first I found myself thinking of wise-ass responses like "you think?" or "you just now figured this out?" But I suppressed the wisecracks, and ended up thanking them for this incredibly relieving news. I can't imagine what it would have been like if they had determined otherwise. To tell the truth, the insurance company has been great to deal with so far.

So it looks like we're moving ahead, though the hospital insists that we keep that Oct. 24 date in pencil. More updates as soon as we have more definite news.

Finally, thank you everybody for all your beautiful cards and notes. Our fireplace is covered with them! While the fire warms our bodies, your good wishes warm our hearts.

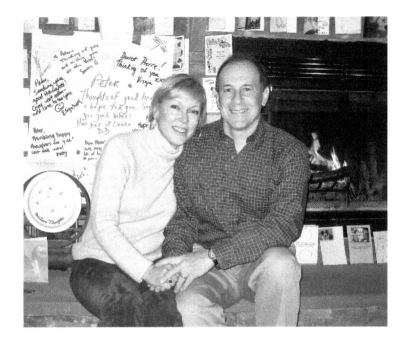

Oct. 16 - Our hospital Orientation Day

On Wednesday, Mary Ann and I had our Orientation Day at Dana Farber. The morning started with a trip to the blood lab, where they drew 23 vials of blood out of me! Luckily I had plenty left, because that was just the beginning of a long day of meetings and tests.

They showed us the radiation area to get a sneak preview of the place I'll get full body radiation treatments – it's sort of like a tanning bed on steroids. Then lots of x-rays, consults with the radiologists, and a quick exam where they poked and prodded all over. Apparently the radiation is going to be a big deal.

I had a pulmonary test, where I got to huff and puff into a little gizmo while watching my breathing patterns displayed on a computer screen. It was fun - like playing a video game with your lungs. Learned I have excellent overall lung capacity, but with some mild constrictions in my inner air passages. Who knew?

My mother then joined us at the hospital so we could all meet with the DFCI social worker. My mother used to be a social worker herself, and it was touching to see how they bonded. It's nice how the Dana Farber team complements their clinical expertise with a deep concern for the more emotional issues, family concerns, etc.

The three of us then met with the head transplant doctor, Dr. Soiffer, which was the highlight of the day. Mary Ann and I had already met Dr. Soiffer, and we were really impressed. I think it was reassuring to my mother to finally meet the guy who'll be taking care of her son, especially because he's such a pleasant, down-to-earth fellow who exudes quiet confidence. (I'm talking about the doctor here, not the son.)

Dr. Soiffer and his assistant walked Mary Ann and me through a million pages of consent forms, explaining each as we signed away. He discussed the various risks and possible side-effects and mortality statistics, calmly and patiently, with a directness that I appreciated. As we wrapped up, he gave me a reassuring wink and said, "You're gonna do fine. See you next week." Wow, for all Dr. Soiffer's medical expertise and accomplishments at one of the world's leading cancer centers, I thought this little gesture was as impressive and powerful as anything. Talk about exuding quiet confidence.

The day ended with me being whisked away for a bone marrow biopsy. As if they didn't get enough blood from me earlier, now they wanted to test my marrow. So they had me lay down on my stomach, they put a surgical dressing over my lower back and upper rear end, numbed the area with some pretty deep shots, then drilled into my hip bone to pull out a sample of my bone marrow. Probably sounds more gruesome than it really was, especially because I've already had several of these procedures and I've gotten used to them. As long as you breathe, stay relaxed, and even chat a bit with the staff, they're not too bad. As I hobbled out to the waiting room to meet Mary Ann and my mother at the end of the long day, they asked how it was. I joked that it was a real "pain in the ass."

Actually, the day was wonderful, and reassuring that I'll be in such great hands. It marked the turning point from months of uncertainty and waiting to concrete action. I like that. They told me that, barring any unexpected complications with the donor, I should be all set to go in on Friday the 24th to start my cure.

Oct. 22 – It's on!

Well now it's finally written in ink, not pencil. The Dana Farber folks called yesterday and confirmed that the donor passed his physical, all their preparations are ready, and I'm confirmed for admission to the hospital on Friday. So here we go.

A rough overview of what's to come: On Friday I'll have minor surgery to install two catheter ports into my chest - these will allow for easy blood draws and infusions without having to start a new IV each time.

On Saturday and Sunday, they'll give me heavy duty chemotherapy to start killing off my blood cells. This will be followed by four days of total body radiation, which will further zap my blood cells.

By Friday the 31st, my blood counts will be nearing zero (and I imagine I'll be feeling crappy). This is when they'll transplant the donor's stem cells into my system via an IV infusion. There's a lot of humor potential there to think that I'll be receiving my transplant on Halloween!

They say I'll feel even more lousy during the second week, before the new blood cells get established. Hopefully they'll take hold and start growing sometime during week three, and by week four my blood counts should start to rise back up again. That's the plan anyway.

I'll have my laptop in the hospital (properly disinfected, of course), and I'll keep you posted with updates from there. I'm not sure how I'll be feeling, but I'll do my best to keep you informed.

Finally, Mary Ann and I again want to thank everyone for your tremendous support. I'll next be in touch from the hospital.

Notes from the present day

OK, I said that I'd interrupt the narrative from time to time with comments from the present day perspective, and I'd like to do so here. Let me share a few things I didn't mention in my blog at the time, but are significant now that I look back.

During that summer of anxiety, one day I went down to our local Social Security office and applied for a disability. I'd already canceled the rest of my year's work, and I knew I'd have a long hospital stay and many months (or more) of recovery ahead. No revenue on the horizon for a long time. Despite the gripes you hear about government bureaucracy, the process moved along smoothly, and the folks at Social Security were great. My case was eventually approved, and they told me to expect small monthly payments after six months of no work. That would end up being a huge source of help to us, in more ways than I could imagine at the time.

Another important thing I did before going into the hospital was to prepare The Pink Folder. I gathered all my financial and insurance records, account numbers, PIN's and passwords, beneficiary information, an advance directive, my will, and other such items, and assembled them neatly into a pink manila folder. Just in case I didn't make it out of the hospital, I wanted to make things as easy as possible for Mary Ann. You might think this was sort of a morbid thing to do, but in fact it was quite the opposite. Both of us appreciated it.

The economy was starting to tumble in the weeks before my hospital admission. Even so, we put down a deposit for a house lot in a new development Mary Ann's employers were planning. It was right on the edge of the National Forest, and we started fantasizing about stepping out our door right onto the cross-country ski trails. That gave us something to look forward to, which was therapeutic in many ways. We also wanted to show her employers some goodwill by helping to start their sales ball rolling. You'd think they would have been delighted to take our deposit, but when we handed the check to Mary Ann's boss, we got nothing back except a strange vibe.

One more special little gesture: Remember that nice September visit by my brother Larry and family? Well his daughter Lily took photos and video clips during the day, and worked them together into a music video. She sent it to me just before I went into the hospital. For the sound track, she chose a great song by one of my favorite bands, U2: "It's a Beautiful Day." It sure was.

Now let's get back to the story in real time. What follows are my blog entries during my hospital stay.

Part 4

THE HOSPITAL STAY

Oct. 25 - Off to a good start

Greetings from the hospital! I've been here a little over 24 hours, and everything is going well so far.

After checking in yesterday I went right to surgery, where they implanted two Hickman catheters in my upper chest. These will be used for the many blood draws and IV infusions I'll be receiving during my stay. The anesthesia they used during surgery didn't knock me out completely, so I was able to listen and even chat a bit with the staff while they performed the procedure. At least I think I was chatting - who knows if I was making any sense. In any case, it was fascinating to hear and feel (painlessly) what they were doing as they threaded two tubes down veins in my lower neck, then popped them out of my chest. I was impressed how they mixed in lighthearted banter with their serious work - real pros.

After the surgery, they wheeled me up to my room. It's a cozy little room sealed off from the hall outside by two sets of doors. I'm in a special ward, further sealed off from the rest of the hospital by several doors, a special HVAC filtration system and so forth. They need to keep everything super sterile in here.

Today I had a nice visit from my parents. Like everyone who comes into my room, they had to get all scrubbed with sanitizer and wear masks and gloves to come in. While they were here, my excellent head nurse Nejor came in and gave me my first dose of chemotherapy. Took about an hour. It felt so benign and peaceful – just like any other IV infusion. But from what I hear, the chemo will soon be brutalizing my insides. This is much more powerful than the palliative stuff I received over the summer up in Littleton. So far no major ill effects, though I hear my stomach won't be too happy after another day of it.

My hospital stay has been pleasant so far - nice quiet comfortable room, great staff, internet access, a TV on the wall in front of my bed, and of course a remote control clicker to switch between all the college football games. Especially looking forward to tonight's clash between Penn State (Mary Ann's alma mater) and the Ohio State Buckeyes. Good luck to the Nittany Lions!

Oct. 27 - Chemo done, radiation underway

Well my two days of high-octane chemo are done. Some brutal upset stomach, but beyond that no problems.

Now here comes the rough part. Today was the first of four consecutive days of Total Body Irradiation (TBI). This will kill off virtually all my existing blood cells, and apparently I'll be in rough shape for a while. Each day consists of two 20-minute treatments six hours apart - reminds me those "double-sessions" pre-season soccer practices many decades ago.

I just got back from my second session today. It's a fascinating process. I had to get all gowned, gloved, and masked up. Then the attendants put me in a wheelchair, covered me with a sheet, and wheeled me through the double doors out of our ward. Though I've been here just a few days, it felt strange to burst through into the "outside," even if that only meant being out in the regular halls of the hospital.

When we approached the crowd waiting by the elevators, the attendant shouted out "Make way, BMT patient!" (That stands for Bone Marrow Transplant.) She shooed everyone out of the way and even kicked the people off the elevator when it arrived, then pushed me onto my own private elevator ride. I guess this is for sanitary reasons - because of my declining immunity, they want to keep me away from others as much as possible. I noticed how cooperative everyone was – or maybe terri-fied. I must have been quite a sight – like a mummy in a wheelchair. They all jumped out of the way almost as if they thought *I* was conta-gious. To tell the truth, I got a kick out of it.

Then the mood gets more foreboding as they wheel you down a maze of hallways deep in the bowels of the building. There's a deep vibrating sound in the background. You go through an incredibly thick door that looks like it could withstand a nuclear blast, then finally into the inner sanctum of the radiation room. They lay you on a slab and put protec-tive shields on specially marked parts of your chest. You just lie there.

The technician who runs the place is excellent – so pleasant and calm. Before he leaves the room, he puts on a CD – what a classy touch to have music playing! For this morning's treatment, it was Michael McDonald singing Motown hits. This afternoon it was Joshua Tree by U2, one of my all-time favorite albums.

Then everyone leaves, the huge door closes with a deep thud, and this massive sun lamp type of thing hanging down from the ceiling rumbles to life.

It's kind of frightening just lying there passively with that contraption rumbling above you, sending waves of radiation into your body. Sort of like being inside a microwave. All kinds of thoughts go through your mind: Apprehension about how sick it will make you; images of those horrible pictures after the Hiroshima bombing; fears about what lies ahead; even worries whether the transplant will work at all and you'll ever get out of here...

You're supposed to lie still, but when U2 starts cranking out "In God's Country," I find my fingers tapping, my fears dissolving into a joyous vision of returning home to Mary Ann and our mountain paradise, renewed resolve and strength running through my body, and a tear trickling down my cheek.

Oct. 28 – Wiped out

I didn't feel much during the first two radiation sessions yesterday, but today – wow, really wiped out. Fatigue beyond fatigue. I slept most of the afternoon. Not a very good host to Mary Ann, who's been staying over at my parents' place in Boston, and our friend Daniel, who stopped by with a surprise visit. Daniel biked over from Cambridge through raw drizzle and horrible traffic – impressive effort! Thanks, my friend.

Three radiation treatments down, five to go. I think I hear the nurse coming in to get me all suited up for my next one.

Oct. 29 - Next to last day of radiation

Third radiation day done. One more left tomorrow, then the transplant the next day.

Getting weaker. Lots of fatigue, upset stomach, brutal diarrhea, some dizziness, and lately dry itchy skin. I'm also losing my appetite. I guess it's going the way it's supposed to. They post my blood counts each day on a white board on the wall near the TV. My counts are on the way down, as intended. I feel it.

Though I might not show it, it's been great to have visitors. Sorry you have to go through all that process with the mask and gloves and sanitizer - also sorry I'm not the most energetic or entertaining of hosts.

Oct. 31 - Day Zero dawns

I had a terrible night last night. Not from the nausea, diarrhea, and pain - I'm getting used to all that. No, it was from unbearable itching. You can't imagine itching could ever feel so bad. I guess the accumulated radiation really dries out the skin, and despite the lotion and drugs they gave me, I had a miserable sleep.

As the night nurse came in this morning to finish up her shift, I asked her to open up the blinds. I wanted to see the first light of dawn coming in today on Day Zero, as they call it - the day of my transplant. As she finished up her shift and was heading out the door, she suddenly stopped and wheeled around and said "Oh, by the way, happy birthday!" It took me a few seconds to realize what she meant, and suddenly the itching didn't seem so bad.

From everything I can tell, all systems go for tonight's transplant. I'll keep you posted as best I can. Happy Halloween!

Nov. 1 – Day One: The morning after my transplant

When I was a kid, I was fascinated by the early NASA space missions. You could say I was a little "space nerd." I even faked being sick once so I could stay home from school and watch one of the launches. I always got a kick out of the way they counted down prior to liftoff ("T minus two minutes," etc.), and then counted upward once the spacecraft blasted off.

Well that's sort of how they time this whole transplant process here. During my first week they marked each day in negative terms (Day

Negative Three, Negative Two, etc.) as we counted down toward the actual transplant. It's now officially the morning of Day One. Of course yesterday was Day Zero, and last night in particular, when I received my new cells, was the moment of "Liftoff."

These blog entries usually flow quite easily for me, but right now I'm struggling to find the words to describe what last night was like - especially all the various emotions involved. Well let me give it a shot.

It was a crazy day around the ward, as many of the staff were wearing Halloween costumes, at least partial ones. During the afternoon and early evening, the excitement started building as we heard little snippets about where my new cells were: They've been harvested from the donor... the plane transporting them is in the air... they've arrived at Logan Airport... they're in the building...

There was a flurry of activity as Nejor prepared the infusion lines, pasted little electrodes all over me, and hooked me up to an additional monitor. I heard commotion out in the hall. My parents and Mary Ann were in the room. We were joined by Matt the hospital chaplain. A second nurse came in to assist, then a third. Someone joked that it seemed like the crowded stateroom scene from the Marx Brothers' "Night at the Opera."

Suddenly Nejor came in holding the cells - a single plastic IV bag of red-pinkish fluid. She cradled the bag in both palms, almost like holding a tiny newborn infant. The nurses did all sorts of checks and double-checks, verbally confirming everything to each other, again reminding me of a NASA mission. As I watched Nejor attach the bag to the IV pole, I felt myself tremble a bit as I thought about what was in that bag and what was about to happen. Chaplain Matt said a nice little blessing, not just for me and my family but also for the donor. Everyone was quiet. My father had to leave the room. I glanced at Mary Ann and saw tears in her eyes. Nejor opened the IV valve, and the cells started dripping into me.

Liftoff.

The rest of the process was rather uneventful - the infusion itself took less than an hour, just like any other IV drip. I didn't feel anything except tired. Mary Ann went outside the room for a little prayer or something with Matt. My father never came back in – I wonder where he went. The nurses kept coming in and out doing their various checks.

Soon things started to settle down, and everyone said good night. When I heard the door click shut for the last time, it didn't take long for all my anxiety, tension, relief, and awe to dissolve into a drug-induced sleep.

Nov. 3 - Here comes the roughest stretch

It's been a few days since the new cells were transplanted into me. I'll always remember that moment when those first few drops of red fluid made their way down the IV tube. But now the emotions have settled down, most of the major procedures are done, and we're into more of a waiting period.

If you'll let me go back to the NASA spacecraft analogy I wrote about before (I promise this is the last time), the period after blast-off is the most stressful and dangerous: The craft shudders, the crew strains against the G-forces, and there's always the risk of something going wrong. It isn't until the engines shut down and the ship glides safely into orbit that everyone can relax.

Well that's sort of the situation we're in here – waiting anxiously to get through the most difficult phase. The chemo and radiation are still churning inside me, continuing to kill off my old blood cells. Meanwhile the newly implanted stem cells are struggling to find their way into my bone marrow. Very few will make it. The doctors tell me that we're entering the roughest part of this journey, and I should expect to feel lousy for the next week or two. What remains unspoken is the uncertainty over whether the new cells will even take hold at all. So all we can do is wait.

But that's OK - this is a normal part of the process. I'd take this type of waiting any day over the anxiety of waiting to find a donor. I'm in great hands here at Dana Farber. (Actually, I'm in the Brigham & Women's Hospital, which is used by DFCI for inpatient care.) Dr. Soiffer and his team are orchestrating every step of the treatment, and it all seems incredibly well organized. You get the feeling they've done this a few times before. The nurses are great, as are the attendants and technicians. Impressive teamwork.

I can't say much for the food – not because it isn't good, but because I can hardly eat anything. Upset stomach, sore constricted throat, no appetite. The only exception is the lactose-free vanilla milkshakes – they're pretty much my sole diet now.

Anyway, once the stem cells get established in my bone marrow, they'll hopefully begin to produce new blood cells. Cancer-free cells. My blood counts will rise, I'll slowly start to feel better, and we can breathe a bit easier. Just like when that spacecraft reaches orbit.

So during the coming week I'll try to add regular updates if I feel up to it. I don't have a lot of energy, so my posts will probably be shorter - which I'm sure most of you readers will probably welcome!

Finally, I'm just blown away by all the comments folks have been adding to this blog. I read every one. Thanks so much for your kind words, good wishes, and prayers.

November 5, 2008 – Election Night

Not much new. I've been feeling really tired lately, drifting in and out of naps all day, and conking out early for the night. Often aided by pills.

94

But last night was an exception. I noticed how excited the hospital staff members were about the election, so I invited them to watch the returns in my room. Apparently there's no TV out in the rest of the ward. Folks kept dropping in all evening, all properly masked and gowned of course. Most of the attendants are from the Caribbean islands, Haiti in particular. I noticed many wearing Obama shirts. My room became sort of like a combination election headquarters and masquerade party, with everyone dropping by with their masks and gowns on. It was a blast. And the excitement kept me awake way past my usual falling asleep time.

Probably most of us remember exactly where we were when various historic events took place. Examples for me include the assassination of JFK, the Apollo moon landing, the Challenger disaster, and the Sept. 11th attacks. Well I can now add one more: I'll never forget lying in my hospital bed, starting to drift off into a drug-induced fog, then hearing the words of Wolf Blitzer saying, "CNN can now confirm that Barack Obama has been elected President of the United States."

Even though I was tired and weak and sleepy, I felt a surge of excitement and pride that our country has come over such a large hurdle, maybe tempered by a deeper sense of foreboding that the toughest part may lie ahead. I wondered if that was true for my situation, too...

Nov. 6 - On the way down

I don't mean to sound alarmist by that title - it's *supposed* to happen. My blood counts are on the way down. They take my blood every morning, send it to the lab, and graph the results on the dry-erase board. The line has been trending downward and is now down close to zero. It's a little scary to see that line way down there.

I'm really feeling it. Fatigue beyond anything I've ever experienced. I could barely lift my laptop from the bedside table to my bed to write this post. Not much of an appetite, except for those milkshakes.

If you want some more of the gory details: sore throat, increasingly constricted; dry mouth; continuing stomach discomfort; skin rashes; diarrhea; weak muscles; and general achiness. Fun.

And if that weren't enough, I just looked down on my pillow and it was covered with hair. I've been looking forward to this part!

But I take comfort in knowing that this is all a normal part of the process. Dr. Soiffer comes in every morning to check on me - usually with a gaggle of residents and med students in tow. He keeps reassuring me that everything is going according to plan. In fact, Soiffer even teased me about it during this morning's visit. In front of his team, he told me "You're doing so well, you're boring." The guy's excellent!

Time passes surprisingly smoothly each day - some TV, some reading, frequent visits from the nurses and attendants, and lots of naps. Apparently I've got a few more days of this. Then we'll hopefully pass another major milestone when my blood counts will start to rise back up. Fingers crossed...

Nov. 8 – A new hair style

Well I'm still in the period where my blood counts are near rock bottom. Even so, I'm feeling relatively OK. Not quite as fatigued as last time. The typical side effects of stomach and digestive problems and skin rashes are still there. Biggest problem is sore mouth and constricted throat - thank god for vanilla shakes. I can't eat anything else.

My hair started falling out the other day, which leaves a mess on the pillow and sheets. So nurse Nejor got some shears and shaved the rest of it off. Still a bit scruffy in the beard, but that should soon be gone, too. I must say I'm pleased with the results - no more bad hair days for a while. What do you viewers think?

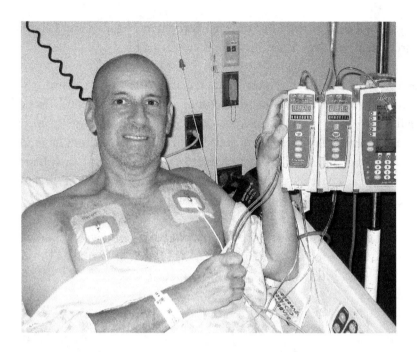

You can also see in the picture my constant companion: the IV pole with pumps and tubes attached. Except for a half hour each day, when they disconnect me to take a shower, I'm hooked up to that thing perpetually day and night. They're always dripping various drugs and fluids into me. You can also see the two tubes poking out of my chest. These are the Hickman catheters I described earlier. They allow for easy infusions and blood draws. Apparently I'll get to keep one as a parting gift when I leave the hospital.

Nov. 9 – Still near the bottom

They tell me these days are the "low point" in the process. All sorts of aches and discomforts and fatigue - but for the most part, tolerable. Days and nights have settled into a routine. I've gotten used to the sounds of the HVAC system, the plumbing, the monitors and IV pumps, the hustle and bustle from the nurses desk outside - in some ways it's all become sort of calming. And when I hear the squeak of the outer door opening, I feel myself perking up a bit.

Before I was admitted, I wasn't sure if I'd be able to have visitors, both because of my sealed-off location and my uncertainty about how I'd be feeling. Well it's been an unexpected pleasure to have visits from family and friends. A piece of me feels bad that all my visitors have to go through such a hassle getting all sanitized and putting masks and gloves on - the other part of me quietly chuckles at how funny everyone looks when they come in. I wonder how I look to them.

Among many great visits, my brothers and sisters-in-law dropped in the other evening with an excellent gift: a DVD of Will Ferrell's "Talladega Nights." Absolutely hilarious, and therapeutic too.

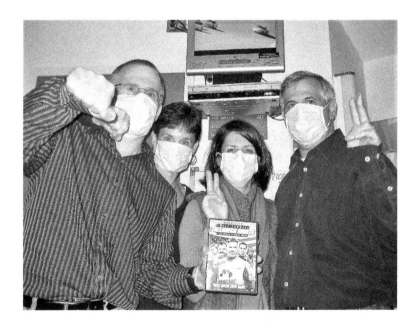

Mary Ann comes down from NH whenever she can. Things are really busy with the real estate work back home, and it's hard for her to get much time off - even for something like this. But somehow she manages, often taking the bus down from Concord after working all day, sleeping on my parents' couch, keeping up a smile. Underneath that smile she looks exhausted. I can only imagine what she must be feeling inside when she sees me like this.

Nov. 10 – Worries and a scare

It's now ten days after my transplant, and I'm beyond the point where they said my blood counts would start to rise. I'm starting to feel nagging worries about whether the transplant will take. Can't do much except wait and stay relaxed. The drugs help.

Many post-transplant patients get fevers, in part because our white blood cells, which fight infections, are so depleted. A fever, and its underlying cause, have to be managed immediately or it can be quite dangerous. Even fatal. Surprisingly, I haven't had a fever - which is partly why the doctors called my case "boring."

Well that changed last night. Enough of being called boring - I decided to liven things up for the staff. I was feeling particularly tired, achy, and crappy, and then I started having brutal chills and uncontrollable shivering. Even though I felt cold, my temperature spiked to 100.7, which is beyond the danger zone for someone in my situation.

So that set in motion a quick chain of events from the whole staff running in and out: additional blood draws, urine sample, lab tests, x-rays, antibiotics and other medications. I was amazed at how calmly and routinely they handled everything.

Anyway, my temperature is now back to normal. I feel better (relatively speaking). Good enough to do one more thing that helps distract me from the worries: reading. Finally finished Lance Armstrong's book called "It's not about the bike - My journey back to life."

Nov. 12 - On the rise!

There have been a few milestones along the way that were especially exciting to write about – for example, they found a donor, we got an admission date, the new cells have been transplanted into me, etc. Well this one just might be the most special of all.

Each day they plot my blood counts on a chart in my room, and for many days the line has been down near the bottom. Yesterday I noticed the reading inched up a bit higher. And then this morning, as the nurse plotted my latest count, he turned around with a little smile. OMG, the reading was way up! The graph line suddenly looked like an airplane soaring upward after take-off. That means my bone marrow is now manufacturing new cells of my own!

To think that that plastic bag of red fluid they dripped into me twelve nights ago is now producing new cells, producing life! A huge sigh of relief, and so much more.

Now not everything has been wonderful. Still many of the same stomach, mouth, throat, and skin problems. Plus one of my catheter lines got badly infected, causing awful pain. They had to pull it out yesterday - for some reason without any anesthetic. Wow, did that hurt! But the good news is that they said I won't need it anymore.

Maybe it's just in my mind, but suddenly all the bothersome side effects don't seem quite so bothersome. After a couple weeks of practically nothing but milkshakes, this morning I suddenly had a craving for a greasy bacon & cheese omelet. Devoured it!

And for the first time, the doctors are even mentioning the "H" word.

Nov. 13 - A look at my world in the hospital

My blood counts continue to rise, and I'm feeling little hints of improvement each day (though still plenty of ill effects). The doctors say I'm doing great. Apparently, I've weathered the treatment better than most, which they attribute to all that exercise in the fresh mountain air.

I thought I'd spend the rest of this entry telling you a little more about the world where I've been cooped up the last three weeks. My room is about 12 x 15 feet at the most. Luckily there's a window with a nice view. Squeezed in front of that are a couple chairs, which I call the "visitors' gallery." There's a tiny bathroom, plus a little vanity counter and sink.

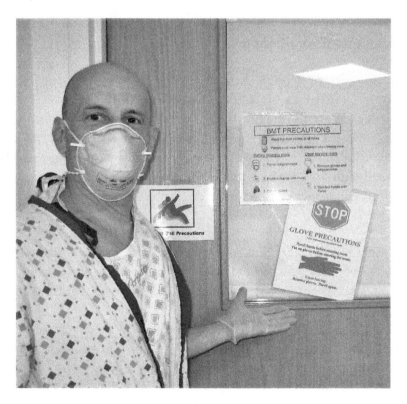

Although I'm usually hooked up to an IV pole, each day I get a little taste of freedom when they disconnect me and prepare me for a shower. Whenever I feel up to it, I use this time to take a short stroll around the neighborhood. I have to put on mask and gloves to leave my room, and I'm restricted to walking laps in about a fifty-foot area in front of the nurses' station outside my door. I can't go beyond that because we're in a restricted, climate-sealed area. Doesn't really matter because that's all I can handle - I'm very weak. The photo shows all the precautions posted before you enter my room.

Well that's a little bit about my world. As nice as it's been in here, I'm really looking forward to leaving the ward and getting outside into the fresh air. It won't be long now, I hope.

Nov. 15 - No place like home!

Well things have happened quickly since my last post! Apparently, my climb out of the low period was unusually fast and robust. Yesterday they did an extra bunch of labs and some physical tests to make sure I'm capable of leaving. My favorite was making sure I can climb stairs. The nurse gowned me up, took me out into the stairwell, and told me to climb a flight. I felt sort of slow and wobbly, but in her view I must have done pretty well because she said "you're good to go."

With that and the other tests, they determined that I'd be ready to leave the hospital today!!! So this morning they began the process of booting me out. Instead of that hideous hospital Johnny gown, I got dressed in my good old blue jeans. My mother had carefully double-washed the clothes I arrived in several weeks ago, and repacked them in sterile zip lock bags - far exceeding hospital cleanliness protocols. It felt great to be wearing real clothes again - and not having to worry about my rear end hanging out!

It was bittersweet saying goodbye to the great staff here. From the doctors to the nurses to the assistants to the technicians and all those others behind the scenes - they all played a role in getting me through this. Despite my weak immune system, there were hugs all around, lots of good wishes, and even a few tears.

And then came that moment when Mary Ann pushed my wheelchair through the hospital door out into the fresh air. I can't describe how wonderful that first breath felt. And how great it was to see my parents waiting with the car, my dad at the wheel ready to head north...

...Three hours later, I'll never forget that first step back into our beautiful mountain home. Mary Ann and her sister had been working their tails off getting the place ready for my return, and it was spotless and sanitary. Gizmo and Miss Peng greeted us, looking a bit confused up at this masked bald headed guy who just entered their world. Doctor's orders are to stay away from the cats for hygienic reasons, but we're going to find that hard.

As I type this, we're relaxing in the living room with my mother, who's staying with us to help out for a while. Just finished dinner - she and Mary Ann had chicken vindaloo, I had baby food. (I can't eat anything except "processed" food for the next few months.) Cats are quarantined in the basement. Wow, what an amazing day. I'm totally exhausted, but working on adrenaline or something. There's sure no place like home.

So I've got a long, slow recovery ahead, and life is going to be quite different for the next few months. More details coming...

Notes from the present day

Before we get back to the story, I'd like to jump back in here with some present-day reflections on my hospital stay. It's amazing what you notice when you look back on things with hindsight.

103

Mary Ann's boss made her work on the day of my admission, so my brother Larry drove all the way up to Bretton Woods to take me down to the hospital. As we were waiting in the check-in lobby, we heard someone say "Code Pink," and all of a sudden all the hospital staff jumped up from their desks and started racing around. All the doors were locked shut, and we were instructed to stay in place. What in the world was going on?

After sitting there for about 45 minutes, we learned that Code Pink meant that a newborn baby was missing from the maternity ward. Everyone immediately scrambled to their pre-determined stations to help seal the hospital and prevent a kidnapping. Well they found the baby, and everything soon returned to normal. I remember being so impressed with how well-planned and efficient the whole event was; it actually gave me some encouragement about the way they'd handle my transplant.

In the years since, unfortunately, I've been reminded of that Code Pink every time there's been a mass shooting or bomb threat at a school. You always see how well trained everyone is these days. Impressive preparations, but also a bit sad – especially when the kids themselves now have to go through the training drills.

Another point about my hospital confinement: I've told you about all the precautions against bacteria, infections, etc. Well the chemo and radiation also destroyed my platelets (the cells that help blood clot), so I was also at high risk for bleeding, external and internal. I wasn't allowed to have any sharp objects in the room, including razor blades. Even the corners of the vanity counter and other furniture were round to prevent bumps and bruises. During one of his early visits when I was still looking scruffy, my father went out and bought me a nice Norelco electric razor so I could shave. I thought that was a helpful gift.

But what I didn't fully realize at the time, it was also a way for him to do something to help. I knew he was very uncomfortable seeing me in that condition, and sometimes he wouldn't even be able to come into the room. Like many men of his generation, he wasn't always comfortable sharing his feelings or discussing things openly.

But I knew he cared, and little gestures like the electric razor were his way of showing it.

A final reflection for now: I'll never forget my release day, especially all the good wishes and (protocol-violating?) hugs with the staff. They were all so wonderful… I don't have too many regrets about how I've handled things during this journey, but one regret is that I didn't go back later and thank them all again.

Now back to the blog, and a whole new adventure: the long, bumpy recovery road.

Part 5

RECOVERY PEAKS AND VALLEYS

Nov. 19 - Slowly recovering at home

Just finishing my fourth day at home. The first few days were rough - I was very fatigued and generally felt lousy (though happy to be home). Spent all but a few minutes lying in bed. I don't even think I had the energy to properly thank Mary Ann and Nancy each time they brought a tray of tea or soup into the bedroom.

Today I can feel myself getting a bit more energy. I was able to sit at the table for a little while and work on a jigsaw puzzle with my mother – very therapeutic. (Can you believe she's 80?) She's been staying with us and doing an amazing job cooking, cleaning, and taking care of me.

I don't know if you can tell from the photo, but the mountains and ski trails are white with snow, and it's starting to look like winter. It won't be long before I'll be able to look out the window and see my ski buddies carving their way down.

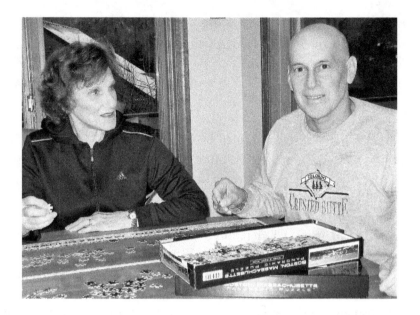

Nov. 22 – It's snowing!

Wow - as I typed the date in the headline above, I just realized that it was exactly 45 years ago almost to this minute when they called us fifth graders in from gym class and told us about the assassination of President Kennedy. One of those historic moments I mentioned earlier that you never forget.

On a lighter note, we woke up today to about a foot of new snow, and it's still coming down. The ski hill across the street is now open, and I've been enjoying watching the skiers slicing through the fresh powder. You'd think I'd be chomping at the bit to get out there with them, but to tell the truth, I'm not. Just holding the binoculars up to the window for a minute or so takes about all the strength I can muster.

With that, I guess what I tried to do this morning was pretty stupid. I got all bundled up and went outside - my first venture outdoors in a month. The windshield wiper on Mary Ann's car has been broken, and I wanted to fix it so she could drive to work. Well that turned out to be a disaster. I was too weak and exhausted even to reach across the hood and grab the wiper blade, let alone get a wrench on it. I ended up brushing off the windshield of *my* car so she could take it instead. Fortunately the snow was light & fluffy. Even so, all I could manage was to brush off just enough so she could see. That wiped me out so much that I had to open the car door and drop into the passenger seat for a rest. By the time I stumbled back inside, I was completely spent - I pretty much collapsed on the mudroom floor, fatigued beyond anything I've ever experienced. It was a humbling slap-down to realize how weak I still am – I guess a valuable reminder of my limitations.

Even so, I did get a good report from the doctor recently. Got all masked up and went down to Dana Farber (thanks to the generosity of neighbors Margaret & Curt, who drove me down and back – 325 miles round trip). Dr. Soiffer said I'm doing very well for three weeks post-transplant, and the fatigue, skin rashes, and stomach problems I'm experiencing are perfectly normal.

And despite my outdoor exertion this morning (maybe even a bit because of it?), I do feel a little stronger this afternoon. I'm noticing that I can stay on my feet longer than before. So I'm heading downstairs to putter around the living room, watch some college football, and continue to work on that jigsaw puzzle.

Nov. 26 - Small signs of progress

Remember my exhausting, unsuccessful attempt a few days ago to fix Mary Ann's windshield wipers? Well today the weather finally cleared, and I ventured outside to try again. It felt great being outside in the fresh air. And this time I got those wipers fixed. Nice to feel I could accomplish something productive.

Came back inside and was a little tired, but nothing like last time. That's a small sign of progress.

Yesterday I passed another milestone of sorts: It was the first day in which I spent more time up and around the house (albeit sitting on the couch a lot) than lying in bed.

Nov. 29 – A step back

They told us that my recovery at home would be a long, slow process, often following a two-steps-forward-one-step-back type of course. Well lately I've taken a step back.

I've had a flare up of what they call Graft vs. Host Disease. This is where my new immune system starts attacking my old cells. This disease can have a wide range of effects, from minor irritant to life threatening. But don't worry - the doctors tell me that my situation is fairly common and manageable with medications. The main outward effects have been skin rashes, upset stomach, headache, dizziness, and fatigue.

One thing that has been impressive (and comforting) has been the way my doctor in Boston stays in such close contact via email. He's constantly monitoring my symptoms, giving advice, and adjusting my medications when necessary. He's a very busy guy, but it's amazing how quickly he always responds to my emails.

I go down to Boston about once a week for doctor visits, blood labs, etc. Sometimes Mary Ann takes me, and sometimes our great neighbors give me rides. Thanks so much! I'll post another update here after my appointment this Monday.

Dec. 4 - Update & Thanksgiving reflection

The news from my latest doctor visit was encouraging. The ups and downs I've been having seem to be under control and getting no worse.

My liver is having some problems, and I still have occasional skin rashes as a result of mild GVH (Graft vs. Host) disease. Even so, I seem to be able to do more and spend more time out of bed and on my feet. Most of my blood counts continue to rise. Most relieving of all, my latest blood test showed zero "blasts," which are the defective cancerous cells that were spreading through my blood before the transplant.

Anyway, it was almost a week ago that I sat down to Thanksgiving dinner with Mary Ann and my mother. I wasn't feeling that well, but in every other way it was about as special a holiday as I could ever dream of. Talk about the true meaning of "thanks giving."

I had so much to be thankful for: For being back home in beautiful Bretton Woods to celebrate my favorite holiday... for being able to get dressed and sit up at a real dinner table... for being able to eat a hearty Thanksgiving meal (courtesy of Omaha Steaks) instead of mushy baby food and milkshakes... and most of all, for the amazing support of these two wonderful women taking care of me.

Thanksgiving also reminded me of that night about five weeks ago when I received the transplant of the new stem cells. Now there was a time to be thankful - for the great hospital staff, for the family members by my side, and for the heroic act of giving by that anonymous donor, wherever he is.

I also recall during that night the hospital chaplain (whom we affectionately dubbed "Matt from Methuen") came in to give a little blessing, and he said something I found particularly meaningful. He talked about the giant sequoia trees in California. Individual sequoias are unable to stay standing during storms, as their mass would topple over in the wind. So they grow in groves, with their roots systems intertwined below ground. This gives them the support and strength to hold each other up during stormy weather. Nice metaphor, eh? (Pretty good for a guy from Methuen!)

So that's something else I'm thankful for: All the support we've received from so many people, in so many different forms. Thanks for the hundreds of cards, emails, and comments on this blog. Even though we can't respond to them all individually, we treasure each one.

We're grateful for the many acts of kindness and generosity: Visiting me in the hospital, giving us rides, shopping for us, dropping off books and DVD's and flowers, and so on. Just calling to check in or offer whatever help we need. So many examples of the best of human nature. One special story: Our friend Johnny G quietly organized a fund raiser to help us with our medical bills – the other morning he drove all the way up from Mass to drop in and surprise us with a check!

Finally, thanks for the wide variety of good wishes and prayers. We've heard that people have offered prayers for us in local Methodist, Baptist, and Catholic churches, among others... a synagogue in New York... a Native American sweat lodge in Vermont.... a Hindu temple in Ohio... with monks in Africa.... and prayer chains in all parts of the country. Mary Ann's father arranged a perpetual membership for me with the Columban Fathers that includes an annual blessing from the Pope... We've received New Age meditations and Reiki healings and Shamanic drum rituals... No matter what outward form these all take, they all come from the same place: the inner goodness of the human heart.

So I understand what Matt the chaplain meant about those sequoia trees. Mary Ann and I have really felt all those roots of support holding us up and helping us through this challenge. And we'll be forever thankful.

Dec. 12 - More signs of progress

When people call these days and ask me how I'm feeling, I often find myself saying "fair to mediocre" or "blah" or something like that. Just being honest.

But you know, when I look at little things from the last few days that would have been inconceivable a couple weeks ago, suddenly I can see tangible signs of progress.

For example, I can now make it up the steps to our second floor without stopping.

The last couple mornings I got out of bed, got dressed, and never returned to the bedroom until evening. Believe it or not, that's a huge step compared to the first three weeks back home. (OK, I do confess to a few naps on the living room couch.)

When I saw the doctor in Boston a few days ago, he said I'm doing well enough that I can come back for my next appointment in *two* weeks instead of one. That was huge!

Today I joined a conference call with my work colleagues. Though I'm far from being able to return to work, it felt great to hear everyone's voice after so many months. Frankly, it felt great to be able to sit through an hour meeting without nodding off.

Last night, I turned the tables on Mary Ann. She's been working real hard at the real estate office. When she came home after work, I was able to prepare hors d'oeuvres and dinner for her, rather than vice versa.

Finally, Mary Ann said that I have "that gleam" back in my eye, and she noticed I'm talking about the future more.

Dec. 18 - Another slide back

Well maybe I got a bit too over-confident (cocky?) in my last post. Or maybe it's just the typical ups and downs to be expected in this long road to recovery. The last few days have seen things slide backward.

Lots of stomach problems and really bad pain, fatigue, light-headedness. Back to spending more of the day lying down.

Went to my local doctor in NH yesterday for some tests. Trying to figure out what's going on with my stomach.

Dec. 23 - A visit to the Emergency Room

Sorry to leave you hanging after my last post. The back sliding I wrote about last time continued for a few days. I kept feeling worse and worse - terrible upset stomach, extreme weakness and fatigue, and rapid weight loss.

Speaking of weight loss, it was especially painful to wash my hands and have my wedding ring slide off my finger into the sink. Grabbed it just in time.

Kept feeling weaker and more miserable - about as sick as I ever imagined a person could be. Agonizing stomach pain. Even worse was that I had no idea what was causing this, or whether it was a sign that my transplant was somehow not working.

By Sunday night I was in rough shape. I vaguely remember Mary Ann by the bedside, asking me questions, taking my temperature, putting a wet face cloth on my forehead. Her voice sounded so far away. I recall drifting in and out of consciousness. I had these weird visions that weren't quite dreams – more like hallucinations? Mary Ann said later I was all curled up in the fetal position, hardly responsive to anything and mumbling "dark thoughts." To tell the truth, I remember wondering if this is what it feels like to be dying.

Although I was too sick to know it at the time, Dr. Soiffer in Boston was monitoring the situation via emails with Mary Ann. When she sent him a particularly descriptive summary of my condition, including my latest temperature, he responded immediately and ordered us to get to the emergency room ASAP. So Mary Ann and my mother and I bundled up and drove through a blizzard to the Littleton Hospital. If you can believe it, I somehow "came to" enough to get dressed and do the driving! I have no idea where I got the strength to do that.

The ER staff were wonderful. Calm, competent, they knew just what to do. They gave me all sorts of tests. It was quite a feeling of déjà vu to be back in a hospital bed with an IV tube sticking into me. After three hours, the ER doc came in and said they'd found the problem. I had a severe bacterial infection in my intestines. Something called Clostridium Difficile. He prescribed an antibiotic that would hopefully take care of it, although it would cause me even more stomach pain for a week or so. Small price to pay.

I still feel lousy physically, but mentally it's encouraging to finally know what was causing the problem, and to be taking action steps to treat it.

A quick post script: Visited the doctor in Boston yesterday, and learned that aside from my intestinal infection, all the blood counts and other measures of overall progress are doing very well. So once I get this infection beat, I should be back on the upswing.

Dec. 31 - Good bye to 2008

The Mt. Washington Hotel had their annual New Year's Eve fireworks tonight. We had a great view looking out our side window - the fireworks were especially beautiful the way they lit up the snowy ground and winter sky.

As we watched the fireworks, we reflected on this crazy year that was about to come to a close.

Exactly one year ago, Mary Ann was just starting to recover from a near-fatal inner ear infection she picked up in China. The ER doctors who saved her said she was 10-12 hours away from death.

That put an end to her international travel, and she soon changed careers, taking a new job with our local resort's realty group. On the day she heard she passed her real estate licensing exam, I was diagnosed with cancer.

June 30th was our one year wedding anniversary. That was also the day I started my first chemotherapy treatment at Littleton Hospital.

As my condition deteriorated over the summer, our greatest source of anxiety was waiting (and hoping) for a bone marrow donor.

When we learned they found a donor in September, it was a joyous relief, followed by more anxiety as we waited to get final confirmation of my admission date.

On Oct. 24, I entered the hospital. On Oct. 31 (Halloween night) I received the transplant of the new stem cells. That was the special moment when my body received new life, and marked the turning point from disease to cure.

I'll always remember the night of Nov. 4, as I watched from my hospital bed the stirring election of Barack Obama. I wonder if that marked a similar turning point for our nation.

On Nov. 15, I came home and began a long period of virtual quarantine. The subsequent holidays marked the ups and downs to be expected in my long recovery - Thanksgiving up, Christmas way down.

The last two weeks of 2008 have been rough – in some way worse than anything I experienced at the hospital. Tomorrow I finish my course of antibiotics for my stomach infection, and hopefully the new year will get off to a better start.

So you can imagine why, as I watched those fireworks tonight, I had all sorts of mixed feelings toward 2008. It was a year filled with indescribable challenges, but also was a year in which both Mary Ann and I had our lives saved. Let's hope 2009 is a bit less eventful.

Happy New Year!

Jan. 13, 2009 - Still struggling... but a success story too

Well I was hoping that 2009 would see things improve, but so far no such luck. Still very weak, tired, shaky, etc. I have been able to do short bursts of activity, but then I have to lie down and rest. What's worse is that I still get occasional stomach discomfort, which terrifies me that my intestinal infection is coming back. I'd pretty much take anything over that.

On the positive side, Mary Ann pulled off a great accomplishment recently. With the cooperation of the National Bone Marrow Program and Mount Washington Resort, she took the initiative to organize a bone marrow drive at our ski area. She had a publicity poster made with my picture on it, and put it up around the ski area. (I always wanted to be a poster child!) The idea was to show me alive and kicking due to the generosity of an anonymous donor out there. Hopefully my story would motivate others to register as donors.

Friends passed the word around. The ski area generously helped with promotions and set up a table. A representative from the National Marrow program came up from Boston to man the table and give out testing kits.

Of course, I couldn't attend, as I'm still quarantined at home. But Mary Ann told me all about it. All told about fifty people got tested and registered - friends, neighbors, employees, total strangers, resort guests. The first person to sign up was the resort CEO who first recruited

116

Mary Ann to work there – that was impressive! He was followed by several other executives from the hotel and resort. A great example of classy management if you ask me.

The rep from the Bone Marrow program told us how unusual it was to have people run a drive *after* they've received their transplant. Usually people do this *beforehand* to help get their own donor. But this was Mary Ann's idea to keep helping others who might need the same gift of life that I was fortunate to receive. I was so proud of her initiative to make this happen, especially in the midst of all her other responsibilities at work and taking care of me.

So maybe I should go back and revise my first sentence above. This event uplifted my spirits, and helped 2009 get off to a good start. Thanks to all who helped, and especially to my wonderful wife.

Jan. 25 - Peach fuzz returning up top

It's been a while since my last entry. And yes, there's no question about it - my hair is starting to grow back. It's had a few false starts before, only to fall out again. But this time seems different. Not exactly a thick rug, more like soft, stringy peach fuzz. Mary Ann's been monitoring the output closely, even examining my head with a flashlight on occasion. We get a kick out of speculating how and where it will grow back - sometimes they say it comes back curlier or greyer. And of course, the big question is will it fill in my previous bald spot?

I hope you realize that this is all just silly banter, and I couldn't care less what happens to my hair.

More important, this is my first blog entry in a long time where I can honestly say I feel better overall. Going up and especially down steps isn't as difficult – I can even jog a few steps. I've been able to spend longer periods without having to lie down and take a nap. I'm becoming more self-sufficient around the house, able to do some cleaning and occasionally preparing dinner for Mary Ann when she gets home from one of her busy days at work. Rumor has it I even drove to the drug store in Littleton by myself yesterday! Yup, it's true – got all masked and gloved up, and ventured out on my big adventure to pick up my own prescriptions. First time driving in three months. (I guess with the exception of that midnight drive through a snowstorm to the ER, which I'm still not sure was real or a hallucination.) It felt fun to drive again, especially because my Subaru has a stick shift.

Yes, my stomach problems are still there, I still get weak and faint, my hands still shake from the drugs, and I have just about zero muscle strength and endurance.

But as soon as I finish this blog post, I'm heading down to the basement to start a new exercise regimen. I'm going to make a little chart of what I do each day to keep myself motivated and on track. I got the idea from the hospital, where they posted my daily blood counts on the wall - I'll never forget how thrilling it was to see them start to rise twelve days after my transplant, marking my return to life. Charts and metrics really help.

Feb. 1 - First time back out on the snow!

OK, so it wasn't skiing. But I did go snow-shoeing the other day. Mary Ann went cross-country skiing, and I decided to tag along with my snow shoes.

I plodded along at a slow but steady pace, while she surged ahead and come back, sort of like a puppy does when you take it for a walk. I surprised myself how far I was able go. We made it up to one of my favorite spots - a hilltop clearing just off the Dark Forest trail, where the whole Presidential Range suddenly opens up right in front of you. I can't begin to describe how fantastic it felt - ninety days after my transplant - to gaze up at that awe-inspiring view, huffing and puffing all that cold fresh air.

Feb. 8 - Day 100!

All the literature and advice you get about recovering from a bone marrow transplant says that the 100th day is a huge milestone. Some of the dietary and other restrictions ease off, and you can breathe a bit easier. (I mean that in a figurative sense, not literally.)

On my 100th day, I'm continuing to feel better. Slowly building up strength and stamina to get back out into the world. Because my immune system is still very weak, I have to wear a mask and gloves when I go out, and avoid close contact with people or any type of germs. I walk slowly, but at least I'm moving.

Just as important as the improvements in my own health, my increased self-sufficiency has finally allowed me to ease the burden on Mary Ann. I think people don't always realize that the strain on the caregiver is far greater than on the patient. Imagine what it's been like for her working 50-60 hours per week in a new job, new career, in lousy economic times, with the pressure of being the sole breadwinner (and health insurance provider)… while her husband has spent much of the last few months lying virtually immobile in bed, often in great discomfort, unable to do most of the household chores. Oh yes, add to all that the fact that his weakened immune system has left him dangerously vulnerable to disease and infection, so the house has to be virtually anti-septic. Can you imagine the pressure that's put on her?

Fortunately, we've been blessed with some great help. In addition to all the generous offers from neighbors, several people have been good enough to come stay with us. It started while I was in the hospital, when Mary Ann's sister came up from Maryland and spent several days working like crazy to scrub every inch of the house spotless. You've heard about all the great help my mother provided by staying with us during the darkest days of my recovery struggles. And recently another of Mary Ann's sisters flew all the way out from San Francisco to spend some time helping around the house, and sharing some much-needed companionship and "chill time" with her sister. Great efforts by all who've come to lend a hand, and more appreciated than we can ever express.

So thanks again to everyone who has helped us get through this difficult first hundred days. I'll keep you posted as we enter the next phase of my recovery.

Feb. 16 - Our first night out together

Valentine's eve was a time to celebrate many things: The 105th day after my transplant, my good bill of health from my recent doctor visit, the feeling that we might just be over the hump. Most of all, just an occasion for us to finally share a night out together.

The doctor said if we're careful about location and food choices, we can now go out to eat. So I made reservations at the fancy dining room at the Mt. Washington Hotel, a fitting place for such a special occasion. I arranged to have a bouquet waiting on the table - not your typical Valentines dark reds, but rather a mixture of white flowers with spring colors.

It was a night of firsts: Our first night out to a restaurant since October. The first time in many months getting dressed up - in fact the first time I'd worn that grey suit since our wedding. My first glass of wine (but don't tell Dr. Soiffer - I think alcohol is still off limits for me). Even something as boring as a plain old salad took on special significance; I hadn't been allowed to eat lettuce or fresh vegetables for well over three months, and that first salad tasted great!

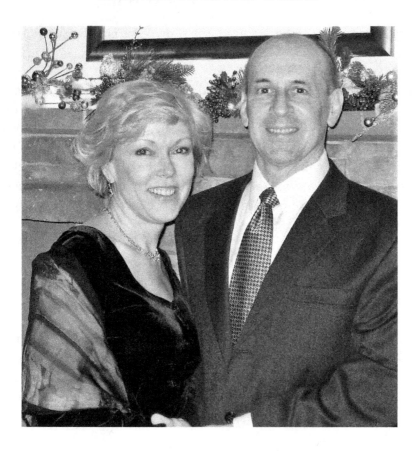

We had the same waitress as for my birthday dinner in October just before I went into the hospital. Even though that was just over four months ago, it seemed a lifetime ago. She remembered us, and welcomed us back warmly. As did several other hotel employees and friends who stopped by our table. And I guess that was the main theme of the whole evening - appreciating how great it was to be welcomed back to living.

Feb. 26 - Back on the slopes!

Well much has happened in the ten days since my last entry. One thing that's happened a lot has been snow - we got five feet in the past week!

In an ironic twist, Mary Ann picked up a bacterial infection and got very sick. It lasted almost a week, and even kept her out of work for four days (which tells you how miserable she was). With my weakened immune system, we had to be very careful I didn't catch her germs. We both wore masks in the house, washed our hands a hundred times a day, slept not only in separate beds but on separate floors, and generally kept our distance from each other. In a bizarre sort of way, it was a bit comical.

Fortunately, she's gotten much better the last few days. And today she was able to join me for one of the most special moments in my whole recovery. Today I decided to try some skiing! We took just a few slow runs on the beginner slope, but it couldn't have been any more wonderful. Saw a bunch of my ski instructor friends who welcomed me back. A half-hour was all my weakened body could handle. As I lugged my skis back to the car, I had to stop and rest about every 15 feet. It's amazing how you can be so thoroughly exhausted, yet exhilarated at the same time.

125 days ago I went into the hospital; 118 days ago I received my transplant of new stem cells; 65 days ago I went to the emergency room thinking I might be dying... I didn't expect to ski this season, and never dreamed I'd be back out on the slopes before the end of February. I'm so thankful I got to experience such unexpected joy today.

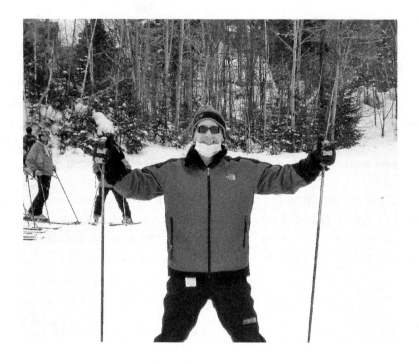

March 1 - News Flash: Mary Ann broke her ankle!

Last night, while bringing pizza into a party she was organizing for real estate prospects at the ski area base, Mary Ann slipped on an icy path and severely hurt her ankle. Fortunately, the ski area staff, various friends and neighbors nearby, and especially the Bretton Woods Ski Patrol all responded heroically. It was clear to all that she had a serious injury - the most amazing thing was that she somehow saved the pizza!

After the patrol got her leg stabilized, they lifted her into the back seat of my car and I drove her to the Littleton Hospital ER. (We're getting a little too familiar with that place.) The staff there determined that her ankle was badly broken in several places, and the orthopedic doctor on duty suggested immediate surgery. They operated last night to put in pins and metal plates. It was really tough saying goodnight as they wheeled her into surgery. What a bummer...

I just got back from visiting Mary Ann this morning in the hospital. She's feeling lots of pain and other discomfort. She had a rough night, especially after the anesthesia wore off. They didn't show her how to use the morphine pump, and she went without any pain killers the whole night. She'll spend a second night there tonight (Sunday), and will probably be discharged tomorrow or Tuesday. She'll be unable to put weight on her foot for six weeks, though they say after a few days she'll be able to hobble around on crutches.

Well this is quite a game changer. I'm relieved that I'm feeling well enough to take care of her, at least to some extent. Thank God this didn't happen a couple months ago – I have no idea what we would have done then. Anyway, I'll update her condition here within a few days.

March 3 - Update

Mary Ann is home from the hospital, resting comfortably, and feeling better overall.

March 7 - A role reversal

Mary Ann has now been home from the hospital for several days. She's set up a nice little "command center" on the bed. She alternates between productive bursts of work and occasional naps when her pain killers kick in.

Fortunately, I'm feeling well enough to take care of her meals and meds and do basic chores around the house. Sort of a role reversal from the past few months.

During surgery, they put in seven screws and a metal plate to hold her ankle together. She'll be unable to put weight on it for a month or two, and she won't be able to drive. So I'll be adding chauffeur to my list of duties. One sad task I plan to do today is to bring home her skis and boots from her locker at the ski area. I'll cherish our few runs on the bunny slope a week ago - the full extent of our skiing together this year.

Once again we've had an amazing outpouring of help from the great Bretton Woods community. Our refrigerator is jammed full of dishes delivered by neighbors. I can't tell you how helpful that is. We have a lot of great cooks around here - even more important, a lot of generous hearts.

March 15 – A birthday and a ski milestone

Mary Ann had a birthday a few days ago. As is all too typical these days, we spent much of her big day dragging ourselves to doctors' appointments - two for her and one for me. She's been feeling better, though still spending most of her time with her leg propped up on the bed, while being surprisingly productive with her work. She struggles with her crutches on stairs. However, she's taken a real liking to the wheelchair some generous neighbors lent us - her technique zipping around the house reminds me of her driving style!

As for me, I continue to feel stronger. I have a touch of guilt about this, but a big milestone the other day was when I went over to the mountain and skied all the way from the top. I still needed to stop and rest along the way, but my technique came back OK. It's hard to describe the thrill of being up there again, seeing that amazing mountain vista, and running into so many friends on the mountain who were totally shocked to see me back up there. I got a kick out of surprising them!

March 23 - More surgery for Mary Ann

Well the challenges just keep on coming. It's been over three weeks since Mary Ann broke her ankle. Frankly it hasn't been healing as well as it should, and we just found out that she'll need another surgery...

Notes from the present day

...And with that, I think I'll interrupt the blog and jump back in with a recap from the present day. Yes, Mary Ann's fall certainly was a game changer, and that opening line from my March 23rd entry turned out to be the understatement of the year. We soon found ourselves caught in a long medical nightmare. Over the next year and a half, Mary Ann would end up having a total of *six* surgeries – four on her ankle, and two more on her knee – all stemming from that fall while delivering pizza.

And the surgeries themselves were the least of it. Not only did she spend most of that period on crutches or in a plastic boot, but it was a time of uncertainty and stress as we bounced from doctor to doctor trying to find a solution, raised hopes followed by crushing setbacks, even eroding faith in the medical profession itself. All this was compounded by increasing problems at her work. And oh yes, I was still stumbling along with my own sometimes rocky recovery journey too! It was a quite a stretch - a real roller coaster ride.

My blog filled up accordingly – post after post chronicling this crazy medical odyssey. So let me condense the story a bit, and summarize some of the highlights (and lowlights) of Mary Ann's orthopedic adventure, and how it intertwined with my own journey. From time to time I'll go back and interweave these summaries around some (but far from all) of my original blog posts, just to bring you back into more of that "in the moment" feeling.

Anyway, the night of Mary Ann's fall, the orthopedic doctor on duty at the Emergency Room was a visiting surgeon from North Carolina. He was up in NH filling in during the weekend. When we asked if he could repair her ankle, he sort of snapped at us, almost as if he felt offended that we would even ask such a question. I still remember his exact words: "Any board-certified surgeon can do that surgery." We didn't know anything other than to take him at his word, so we said sure, go ahead. Big mistake on our part. Although we had no idea at the time, our orthopedic nightmare had just begun.

After the surgery, Mary Ann suffered through a miserable night without any pain killers - the night nurse never trained her properly how to use the morphine pump. In the morning, the surgeon checked on her briefly, said everything went fine, and then flew home to North Carolina. We never heard from him again. A couple local orthopedic docs soon stopped into her hospital room; it was odd how they seemed to be vying for who got her as a patient. She finally ended up with one (to whom I'll give the pseudonym Dr. Indecisive), and he took over her case. After a couple days in the hospital, he sent her home, saying that she'd be fine after a few weeks on crutches.

But Mary Ann's ankle pain kept getting worse, not better. We tried to go back to Dr. Indecisive, but for some reason he was unable to see her. (I can't remember exactly why.) Her pain got so bad that we ended up going to the Emergency Room. This time there was another visiting orthopedic doc on duty, a very nice young fellow from upstate New York, just starting out on his career. After he examined her ankle and the x-rays, he did something I'll never forget: He closed the curtain around her bed, pulled us in close, and whispered to us that the surgery had not been done well, and her ankle was not healing properly. I don't know if that violated any type of medical protocol, but his candor sure ended up being valuable to us.

We eventually went back to Dr. Indecisive, and he lived up to his pseudonym as he hemmed and hawed over her latest x-rays. We practically had to prod him into doing a second surgery. We didn't know any better at the time, but in hindsight we should have read the signals more clearly. In any case, he did the surgery, and Mary Ann was soon zipping around on her crutches. It appeared she was finally on the road to recovery.

So I decided the time was right for me to take an important recovery step of my own. Let me return you the blog for a while to tell the next phase of our story in real time. As you'll see, the roller coaster ride was just getting started.

April 12 - On my way to Florida

Hello! I realize it's been a while since my last post, and occasionally people say they worry if they don't see an update.

In a nutshell, both Mary Ann and I are doing better. We took a little stroll today, our first time outside together in nice weather since October. She moves along well on her crutches. She's been cleared to return to work part-time at the real estate office, though after several hours in a sitting position her leg really hurts. So she still spends a good chunk of the day working from home with her leg elevated. She gets a lot done from either location.

She's also well enough that, with a full refrigerator and some friends scheduled to come over to help take care of her, I can leave for a few days. I recently received clearance from my cancer doctor to fly, so tomorrow I'll be heading down for a long-overdue trip to see my parents in Florida. It'll be a big step in returning to normalcy.

April 18 - A special trip

Up until a few days ago, the last time my parents saw me was in the depths of winter, when I had just started to climb out of my lowest, darkest period. I was still emaciated, weak, and bald, but at least I was starting to recover enough for them to feel comfortable to take their annual trek to Florida.

So a few days ago I took my first airplane trip in ten months (itself a significant milestone), and flew down to visit them. I rubbed on a ton of hand sanitizer and kept my mask on tightly the whole way. I felt fine, though people looked at me funny. As I exited the plane and walked through the terminal in Orlando, I felt a little extra bounce in my step as I neared the place my parents would be waiting. I knew they'd be pleased with how much I'd improved since they last saw me.

And sure enough, I could tell they were thrilled when they saw me. It was a special reunion, as you can imagine.

The few days down there were relaxing and wonderful. I know my parents were relieved to see me on the road back to health. Just sitting around the breakfast table, sipping coffee (and awesome fresh squeezed juice from oranges picked right down the street), reading the newspaper, watching TV, hanging out, strolling in the warm sun, swimming, even hitting a few tennis balls... Every one of those little mundane moments couldn't have been any more meaningful.

I'm back in New Hampshire now, where I've noticed a few crocuses poking up, and continuing signs of our area coming back to life after the long, snowy winter. Still glowing from a great visit with my parents. Mary Ann managed fine while I was gone. Her next day off we're thinking of getting out and taking a little road trip out into the world again.

April 21 – Bob Gordon, 1924-2009

My father died suddenly yesterday. When my mother found him, he was sitting in a lounge chair by the pool, his book still open in his hands. The same chair he used after our swim together a few days ago. As crushed as I am, I'm gratified that it was quick and without suffering.

When I heard the news, my first reaction was shock. A couple seconds later I thanked God that I had the chance to see him last week, and even more important, that he had the chance to see me. As I tried to express in my previous post, there was just something special about that visit - sort of a sense of everything settling comfortably back into place. I know how deeply it touched him to see me looking so much better - and I know that knowledge helped give him peace as he left us yesterday.

My mother seems to be holding up well. My deepest thanks to those who've already reached out to support her through this. I'm on my way back down to Florida today to help her with arrangements. My brothers will be joining us down there, and we'll all make our way back north at some point soon.

PS - Something amazing just happened. It's a cold, raw dawn as I'm typing this - there's sleet in the air. As I finished typing the last sentence above and was just about to "publish" this post, I looked out at the mountains across the way, with the ski trails still covered in snow. Suddenly, for about ten seconds, there appeared a rainbow.

April 27 – Back from Florida

Back from a whirlwind trip to Florida. My brothers and I flew down to be with my mother and help her take care of things. We shared all sorts of memories, emotions, and yes - even lots of laughter.

Got her back up to her apartment in Boston, where she's settling in well and getting adjusted to life alone. I know it's going to be a long process, especially after the shock and grieving wear off, and reality sets in.

May 7 - Four healings intertwined

Much has happened since my last post, all different ways of moving forward. Yesterday Mary Ann had an appointment with her orthopedic doctor to check out her ankle. We were both anxiously hoping for good news, but quietly fearing disappointment based on the way things have been going for us lately. What a relief to hear the doc say it's healing well, and that she could abandon the plastic boot and resume normal activity. Mary Ann bounded out of that office with more excitement than I've seen from her in months, spouting quotes from Martin Luther King: "free at last, free at last!"

Speaking of doctor's appointments, I recently got a great report from Dana Farber. My blood counts are all back to normal levels, with the exception of my red blood cells and liver functions. They assure me this is normal. Just as encouraging, I picked up a head cold recently and generously decided to share it with Mary Ann. I fought it off after a couple days, while it whacked her harder than me. Though I hated to see her suffer, this shows that at least part of my immune system seems to be working - a few months ago that cold could have had much worse consequences.

The loss of our father has brought my brothers and me together in some surprisingly pleasant ways. Along with our usual banter and wise cracks, we've had some nice conversations about the best way to memorialize his passing. We divided up his ashes so we could dispose of them in our own individual ways, but we also wanted to do something jointly. So we all met in the little town of Lincoln where we grew up, and buried some of his ashes under a tree near the little league baseball field where he spent so many hours watching us all play. Our way of saying thanks to the great childhood he helped provide to us.

Down in Boston, my mother seems to be adjusting to her new life alone. After living with someone for 59 years, it must be difficult to get used to the quiet, the empty space, the changes in life's mundane routines. It's a slow healing process that cannot be pushed, with many ups and downs along the way. She appears to be handling it well, thanks in part to the great support of family and friends.

May 15 - The most amazing gift

Yesterday I received a wonderful surprise visit from Nancy, one of my work colleagues. She drove all the way up from Mass. I hadn't seen her or any of my other work associates in a year.

Nancy brought me a gift that blew me away. It's something called a Senbazuru. It's a spectacular mobile consisting of a thousand, multi-colored origami cranes. Japanese tradition says this helps a person recover from illness.

Apparently the whole group down there started making this last summer, after they heard of my dire diagnosis. They taught each other how to fold these little paper birds, and they'd make a few at a time when they could find a few minutes in the lunchroom or at home.

Yesterday, when Nancy showed up, was the first I ever saw or even heard about this amazing gift. As you can imagine, it touched me deeply.

What an incredible gesture - like so many episodes from this journey, another reminder of how wonderful the human spirit can be. And even though I wasn't consciously aware of it until yesterday, I know this Senbazuru lived up to its tradition by helping me make it through the fall and winter.

Anyway, spring has come to the mountains, life is moving forward, and I think I'm nearing the end of this blog. Maybe another couple entries, and then it'll be time to wrap it up. Thanks for following along. Stay tuned.

May 27 – Medical updates: My next-to-last post

Things are moving along well, so barring some unexpected developments, this will be my next-to-last post. I thought I'd give a medical update, and maybe answer a few questions you've been thinking about.

Overall I'm doing much better. More energy, more strength, more stamina, more hair. Tomorrow I have my first haircut in eight months! I take fewer naps. A couple days ago I went for a hike with my neighbor Daniel, and we ended up on top of Mt. Willard, my first real summit since last summer. People keep telling me I look good. (Funny, they never said that when I was healthy.) My blood tests continue to be OK if not perfect.

So what are my risks? My immune system is partially recovered, but I'm still at risk for germs, infections, etc. I still wash my hands a lot with anti-bacterial soap, and I still wear a mask if I'm in a crowded situation. I can't eat raw meat or sushi for the rest of my life - not a great loss as far as I'm concerned.

Another risk is Graft-vs-Host Disease (GVHD). So far I've made it safely through the short-term GVH period with relatively mild side effects. I'm taking all sorts of pills every day to manage this, including one that partially suppresses my immune system. The biggest effect of my GVHD has been dry, scratchy eyes – apparently my body can't produce tears anymore. Ironic, eh?

I also have elevated risk of other types of cancers popping up. Not much I can do about that except keep on monitoring things closely.

You might be wondering whether my leukemia has any chance of returning. As far as I can tell, that's possible but unlikely. There have been no signs of any cancerous blood cells. The transplanted stem cells seem to have taken hold in my marrow and are continuing to produce normal healthy cells. Last doctor's visit I even found out that I've changed blood types! Go figure that!

Well this is starting to sound like one of those season-ending TV shows where they try to build up to a big finale. I hope I can live up to it. See you next time for my last post.

June 2 - No, not my final post - Mary Ann needs more surgery!

Well, I thought life was settling back into place enough for me to wrap up this blog, but no such luck. Unfortunately we got thrown another medical curveball today, so no grand finale for a while.

Though Mary Ann has been walking and moving around better, she's also been feeling more and more pain lately. Something just hasn't been right, and frankly her foot has been looking increasingly misshapen. So today we went back to her orthopedic doc. After some prodding from us, he admitted that his surgery wasn't healing well, so she'll need another surgery - her third!

This was a devastating jolt to us. It's not so much the surgery itself, but the return to square one, the weeks of immobility, the cast and crutches all over again... not to mention the setback to her work at a very difficult time. Things have been getting tougher over at the real estate office, and I don't think it's just the slow economy.

For over a year my wife has been an absolute pillar of strength. Well today she broke down and sobbed. We both fell into a round of "What have we done to deserve all this" self-pity. And neither of us tried to talk the other one into feeling any differently.

So this adventure continues...

Part 6

THE CLIMB OUT

Notes from the present day

When I look back on that last post, even now many years later, my heart sinks. We had suddenly tumbled back down into one of our deepest valleys. Here I'd come back so far with my own recovery, and now this. We started wondering about the unfairness of it all, whether we were cursed in some way.

We'd lost confidence in Dr. Indecisive, but had no idea where else to go. It was an awful feeling of uncertainty. We felt cynicism and mistrust creeping in. The only antidote was to take action, so we started networking around for other options.

We found our way to a foot doctor at New England Baptist Hospital in Boston, a place so renowned for orthopedic expertise that many of the Red Sox and Celtics players went there. The doc examined Mary Ann's ankle, took one look at her x-rays, and could barely maintain his professional composure. He blurted out that he was "pissed to see shoddy work like that!" Good for him for being so candid!

Apparently, neither surgeon had repaired Mary Ann's ankle properly, and now it was a mangled, increasingly deformed mess. The doc was ticked off that they'd cleared her to walk. No wonder she'd been having such pain! He immediately ordered her back onto crutches.

In another refreshing bit of candor, he admitted he didn't feel confident he or his colleagues could do the repair themselves. Fortunately (if anything can be "fortunate" about this whole episode), he referred us to a highly-regarded surgeon at a competing hospital in Boston who was a trauma specialist, and an expert in repairing botched surgeries.

We made our way over to the hospital where this guy worked. I'll give him the pseudonym Dr. Trauma. He squeezed us in for a quick consult in between surgeries – he was still wearing his surgical scrubs. No chit chat or pleasantries – he got right down to business as he checked out Mary Ann's ankle. When we came back a few days later to discuss the next steps, Dr. Trauma strode in right past us and put something up on the x-ray display. It was a meticulously detailed diagram of his surgical plan. We were blown away. The guy might not have had the warmest manner, but what focus and preparation! We were sold. We agreed to the surgery, which he scheduled for later in June.

Dr. Trauma cautioned us that Mary Ann would not only have to remain on crutches for three months after the surgery, but she could put no weight on her ankle for the whole time. "Absolutely zero weight. That's non-negotiable." He was a tough, straight shooter, but we liked his style! As we left the appointment, I remember thinking there goes another summer of hiking together...

An interesting sidelight: Dr. Trauma worked at an inner-city hospital in what I guess you could tactfully say was "not the best of neighborhoods." But apparently it was a great location for him to practice his specialty repairing damage from falls, fights, and gunshot wounds! The waiting area was like a combination war zone and circus. Patients on wheelchairs and gurneys strewn all over, with every manner of injury and disfigurement you could imagine. Teenage gang-bangers; injured athletes; sweet little old ladies wearing fancy hats; occasionally even prisoners wearing orange jumpsuits in shackles & chains accompanied by armed guards! Once Mary Ann overheard a patient boasting that she'd sold her pain medication on the street for $20 a pill. You get the picture. Quite a change of scenery from our remote, lily-white world up north – and we loved it!

Anyway, I think it must be pretty clear by now that my cancer story branched out in many directions far beyond my own treatment and recovery. I assume that's also the case for many others. Life goes on in all its multi-faceted ways, and the cancer journey inexorably intertwines with it. You can't separate the two. So let me return to the blog for a while, and I think you'll see a little more of what I mean.

June 21 - Father's Day reflections

I was in the drug store the other day picking up my prescriptions. As I walked past the greeting card section, there was a sign reminding shoppers to buy their Father's Day cards. For a brief second, I caught myself thinking *"Oh, I should pick up a card,"* and then it hit me...

It was exactly two months ago today when Bob died. (That's what we called my father.) I haven't written much about him in recent entries, as Mary Ann and I have been going through all sorts of challenges of our own. But under the surface, the grieving and healing process has continued, often intertwining with our own ups and downs. A combination of nostalgia, occasional sadness, and a surprising amount of humor and warmth. At times my father was a difficult man, but lately we've been feeling a growing sense of respect for the goodness of his heart.

We've found ourselves playfully imitating some of his quirky mannerisms, like the way he'd throw up his hands in exasperation and exclaim "it's over" when the Red Sox fell a run behind in the second inning. Or the last words I ever heard him say as he dropped me off at the airport after my April visit: "Come back down soon, and next time bring Peg Leg." Yes, he was a colorful character. And we've found humor a great way both to soothe the pain of his loss, and keep the warmth of his spirit living on.

Which leads to one particularly heart-warming story. To help my mother dispose of Bob's belongings, I took some of his clothes. He was a snappy dresser, and among other things, I took a very nice pair of his cashmere-lined leather gloves.

A couple weeks ago, Mary Ann and I were hanging out in the living room when, to our horror, we saw our cat Gizmo dragging one of Bob's expensive gloves down the steps. Our first reaction was to yell sharply at him to "drop that glove!" Gizmo did so and scampered up the stairs. But a little while later he came back down with the other glove in his mouth, and dropped it gently at my feet. We just shook our heads and laughed. Gizmo's gesture was such a sweet way of honoring Bob and warming our hearts. The gloves have become his favorite possession - he treats them with such reverence as he drags them around the house. How can you do anything but smile.

In the last few weeks, I buried some of Bob's ashes near the beginning of the Greenleaf Trail up Mt. Lafayette, where he took me on my first big mountain hike 45 years ago; I also buried some at the top of tiny Elephant's Head, the last "peak" we ever climbed together. I thought that would make a nice kind of symmetry.

Mary Ann knew Bob for less than four years, but they developed a great bond. She took some of his ashes and sprinkled them in secret locations around the Mt. Washington Hotel, a place he loved.

And today, Father's Day, I thought would be an appropriate time to bury the last of his ashes. I decided on a hidden spot out in the woods near our townhouse, a quiet, reflective place we call our meditation garden. Mary Ann couldn't manage her crutches on the rugged path to get out there, so she tossed them aside and actually crawled on hands and knees! We got to the spot behind a huge boulder. I dug a hole, poured his ashes in, then filled the hole and covered it with a rock. I noticed a feather nearby, so I stuck it in the ground as a marker, along with a couple sticks. As I finished the little memorial, I turned to notice

138

that Mary Ann was crying. She loved Bob. When we got back inside our house, I thanked her for her tears.

June 24 – Mary Ann's surgery moved up to tomorrow!

We just got notified that the surgeon had an unexpected opening in his schedule tomorrow, so we're heading down to Boston. I'll keep you updated from the hospital.

June 25 – PM update from the hospital

I'm writing this from the hospital in Boston. According to the doctor, Mary Ann's ankle surgery went well this morning. It was extremely complex, and took almost three hours!

She's still having pain and nausea, but it's starting to decline. She's looking a lot better the last couple hours - in fact she even let me take and post this photo. She made me promise not to show the bucket on the floor.

See the teddy bear? That's a little tradition we started when she was hospitalized a few years ago with that inner ear infection. That night it tore my heart out to have to leave her alone in the hospital, so I ran out to the shop and got her a little toy creature to cuddle up with. You might think that's sort of silly for grown adults, but we don't - we've been doing that ever since.

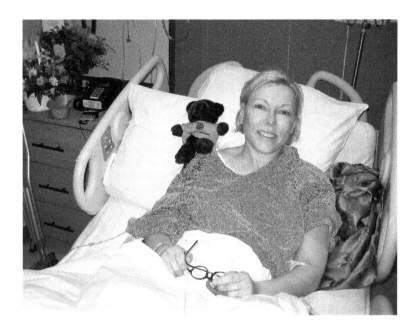

Mary Ann's room has become increasingly popular the last hour or so, as the news about Michael Jackson's death has been spreading around the hospital. Nurses and attendants have been stopping in to check the latest on our TV. Reminds me of election night last November, when my hospital room suddenly became a popular drop-in spot for the staff.

Mary Ann has been doing well enough the last hour or so that they took her down for some more tests. And guess what? You're not going to believe this, but they just wheeled her back from an MRI on her *knee*! It's been painful and swollen lately, and the ankle surgeon was concerned enough to order the MRI. He thinks she damaged the knee as well as her ankle in her fall. OMG, what's gonna come next?

Anyway, when Mary Ann temporarily "came to" a while ago, she picked up her cell phone and snuck in a quick call. (Cell phones are not allowed on the ward, although we've gotten the nurses and attendants to promise they won't bust us.) In the midst of her morphine &

oxycodone stupor, she had the concern to call her work colleagues to check on a big real estate sale that was hopefully going to close today. And apparently it did!

But that's only part of the story. It struck me that when she first broke her ankle back on February 28 to start this whole nightmare, she was working on this *very same sale!* She'd arranged a pizza party that night to introduce some potential home buyers and their kids to some local homeowners' families. She slipped on an icy path while schlepping pizzas to the party.

That night in the Littleton Hospital emergency room, as they were prepping her for emergency surgery, she grabbed her cell phone and somehow managed a quick call to make sure a follow-up appointment she had with these buyers the next morning would be covered by someone else. And guess what – those were the same buyers who finally closed on their purchase *today*, almost four months later!

I hope you'll pardon this little bit of cheerleading for my wife – her sales creativity, passion, and persistence continue to amaze me every day.

Notes from the present day

Every time I hear a Michael Jackson song, I think back to the bustling scene in that hospital room. While the world lost a great performer, that was the day Mary Ann's fortunes finally changed for the better (at least with her ankle). Dr. T got it right. His brilliant surgery not only repaired her ankle, but eased a huge burden of stress and anxiety on us.

As I look back on that blog entry – especially the part about Mary Ann's sales efforts - it also reminds me of something I didn't mention then but can now say freely. Way back when she planned that pizza party, her boss was very resistant to the idea. In fact, she made Mary Ann pay for the pizza out of her own pocket! That was typical - it seemed they tried to stifle every idea she had, almost as if in some odd way they were trying *not* to sell real estate. Something strange was going on there...

Lots happened over that summer of my Year One, so let me give a brief recap. I had a huge milestone in my own recovery. In August, I returned to work part-time (*very* part-time), and led my first workshop in well over a year! It went great. I was exhausted, but nobody knew. It would take a while to build up the stamina to return to a normal work and travel schedule, but it felt great to get that first one under my belt.

Mary Ann's ankle kept feeling better, though she didn't dare violate Dr. Trauma's orders to keep all weight off it. She followed his orders to the letter.

The big real estate development at our resort eventually sputtered to a halt, and Mary Ann's position was eliminated. She was reassigned to handling resales of existing resort condos, which in those tough economic times was like working in a shark tank. It didn't help that she was on crutches.

Meanwhile her knee did turn out to have damage from the fall, and we started looking for the right doctor to fix it. We had a disheartening feeling of déjà vu as we searched around, but at least we'd learned our lesson and didn't just settle on the first surgeon who came along. In one case, we drove all the way down to Boston (three hours) to see a knee doctor somebody recommended to us. The guy barely looked at Mary Ann's knee or x-rays, and he ended the visit with one of those let's-do-nothing-for-a-while type of brush-offs. As we left, we overheard him dictating his notes, which included the phrase "typical middle aged woman." Ouch.

We finally found a knee surgeon up near home who worked for the US ski team. Great guy, totally competent, excellent reputation - we felt we'd be in good hands when it was time to turn to her knee.

Overall, my health issues were still there, but they weren't dominating everything the way they had. I was more focused on helping Mary Ann, as well as rebuilding my own life back toward normal. As I look back over my blog posts in this period, I notice that they became less of a chronicle of my medical ups and downs, and more contemplative toward other things. You'll see what I mean as I take you back to my blog now.

Sept. 2, 2009 - Senator Kennedy, the HR office, and the healthcare debate

The other day we ended up glued to the TV watching the funeral and burial of Senator Kennedy. Tremendous people watching, especially if you like politics. Very moving. Inspiring. Historic. And surprisingly educational.

Why educational? Well one of the things I like about Mary Ann is her voracious appetite for reading, for learning, for Google-searching and finding out stuff. And rather than just tossing ill-informed opinions around, as so many people seem to be doing these days, she went to work researching the substance behind Senator Kennedy's work in the senate.

Now, as background you should know that she comes from a conservative Omaha family. Mary Ann herself was once a dedicated member of the Young Republicans Club, and like many of her colleagues, she had a negative opinion of Kennedy. But through her research, both of us have been able to cut through all the rhetoric and learn a lot about the senator from my native state.

Having grown up in Massachusetts, it felt like Kennedy had *always* been our senator. (In fact he had since I was nine years old.) In some ways maybe we took him for granted, or even wrote him off as a left-over relic from an out-of-date ideology. Over the years, I've often criticized his personal life or joined in as people made jokes at his expense. But somewhere deep down, I've always believed he worked sincerely for the good of everyday folks like us. Well we never appreciated how much until the last few days. Here's why:

There's a little post office in the Mt. Washington Hotel where we get our mail. Down the hall there's also a Human Resources office for resort employees. You access both from a little side door near the parking lot, far from the grandeur of the main entrance. The other day we had business in both places, so I drove Mary Ann over, and used our temporary handicapped permit to park in the handicapped space so she didn't have to hobble too far on her crutches.

There are some steep steps up to the side door, and also a handicapped ramp off to the side. Unless you need it, you probably never even notice the ramp. But try being on crutches for six months (or living with someone who is), and you certainly appreciate it. Mary Ann has found stairs to be especially difficult and dangerous, so those ramps are a godsend. And you know who was one of the main driving forces behind the Americans with Disabilities Act that made these things so pervasive? Senator Kennedy.

As we went into the HR office, I noticed a bulletin board with several employment posters on it. One of them was about anti-discrimination laws. I was reminded that Kennedy was long a fighter for laws banning discrimination in the workplace. And you could see the results all around us in the rich diversity of the hotel employees coming and going through the bustling hallway. Come to think of it, Mary Ann I were both getting to the age where many employers might be tempted to discriminate against *us!*

Nearby was another poster stating the minimum wage requirements. The minimum wage is still so low it's almost laughable - on second thought, no, not really, because there's nothing funny about working full time and bringing home an income below the poverty level. In fact it's an embarrassment in our nation, the "wealthiest" on earth. But at least there *is* a minimum wage, and it's been raised begrudgingly over the past few decades. And during that time the loudest voice constantly bellowing out in support of a humane minimum wage has been Senator Kennedy's.

144

So there we were in the Human Resources office as I filled out the paperwork to switch over my health insurance coverage from the COBRA plan I'd been on to Mary Ann's current plan with the resort. If you don't know what COBRA is, it's basically a law that allows anyone who leaves or loses a job to continue purchasing that employer's health coverage for a designated period. For someone who is caught between jobs, it can be a life saver. And I mean that almost literally. For the past 17 months, my medical bills have been well over a half-million dollars, and thank God most of that was covered through my COBRA plan. By the way, one of the most instrumental leaders behind COBRA legislation, and the security it provides workers in an unstable workplace? Ted Kennedy.

Anyway, we completed our paperwork at the HR office, much to my relief. When we came home, the phone rang and it was my mother, calling to catch up. She's been doing well adjusting to widowhood, though still struggling to straighten out things with my late father's estate - the complexities of Florida probate law have been confusing and overwhelming. However, she said that at least her health coverage was dependable, convenient, and a source of comfort. Yes, she's on Medicare - another one of those "big government programs" that people like to bash, but no senior could do without. And another accomplishment in the amazing legacy of Senator Kennedy.

Now as appreciative as I've been toward my own health care coverage, what you might not know is how close we came to disaster during the past couple years of major job and life changes. We're relatively knowledgeable about the intricacies of the insurance system and how to play the game to avoid a lapse in coverage. But even so, due to a few minor oversights, I came within a wink of letting my policy expire. And if that happened, I guess we'd either have faced financial ruin or I wouldn't be alive anymore. Why? Well do you think I'd ever have a chance of getting insurance ever again with leukemia as a pre-existing condition? Not under the current health care system. And people don't think it needs to be changed? For years (way before Obama even came onto the radar), Kennedy has been crying out for portability of coverage, and the elimination of pre-existing conditions as a disqualifier.

And pre-existing conditions aside, what about people who are out of work, or whose coverage has lapsed, or the self-employed, or those who work for a small business that can't afford to provide coverage? Have you ever tried to buy insurance as an individual? It's a horrible deal, with huge deductibles, outrageous premiums, and hardly any coverage for anything. Mary Ann and I have both been pondering starting up our own businesses. The greatest barrier? Getting reasonable health care coverage. It's almost impossible as an individual. Think of how this is stifling small business and entrepreneurship and innovation.

Senator Kennedy has been crying out for health care reform for decades. He made great strides in this area, but almost to his dying breath was constantly calling out for more. He certainly had flaws in his private life, but he showed (much like ex-President Bush) the admirable ability to turn his life around. And in his heart, I truly believe he cared for something that has gotten obscured by all the partisanship and fear-mongering in our politics recently: The simple belief that in this wonderful country, all people should have an opportunity to lead a life of security and dignity.

As we watched Senator Kennedy's burial, I could tell that Mary Ann was visibly moved. She's made a 180-degree change in her opinion of him recently. It's hard not to when you experience what we've been through, and realize the many tangible ways that our lives have been touched by his efforts. Thanks, Ted!

Sept. 14 - A time to give back

First, a quick medical update. I had my monthly appointment last week, and the findings were mixed, although the overall trend is still good. My liver readings are still off, which means my one-drink limit will be moved down to zero for a while. No big deal.

Mary Ann had an encouraging check-up with her ankle surgeon. Her ankle continues to heal well, and she has surprisingly good range of motion. He cleared her to start putting weight on it in six more days! After almost seven months of absolutely no weight on it (except for a couple painful weeks of ill-advised doctor's orders in May), this is going to be a huge moment for us. Mary Ann even said she's going to wake up and test her ankle at *one minute past midnight* on the appointed day!

———※———

Despite all the medical challenges we've gone through (and maybe because of them), Mary Ann and I have tried to find ways to reach out and help others. A few nights ago we were invited to speak during evening services at the local synagogue in Bethlehem. We told our story, focusing on spreading awareness of the "Gift of Life" bone marrow donor program for people of Jewish heritage. That's where I got my donor from. (Bone marrow donation is one of the places where ethnicity really does matter – your best chance of finding a matching donor is from someone of similar ethnic ancestry.) We were warmly received by the congregation. I've never been much of a church or synagogue goer, but I have to say it ended up being a special, rewarding evening.

You might remember that last January Mary Ann organized a very successful bone marrow donor drive "in my honor" at our ski area. I was too weak and sick to attend. But this week, she's arranged a similar appearance for both of us at a local health fair. We'll have a table, literature, and testing kits to encourage people of all backgrounds to join the National Marrow Donor Registry. I'm so thrilled I'll be able to join her this time, and to offer myself as an example of someone who's been blessed with renewed life through the generosity of an anonymous donor. It's the least we can do to spread the word, and maybe help someone who's in the same shoes we were in a little over a year ago.

Sept. 25 – That's one small step for woman...

Mary Ann's ankle surgeon is a no-nonsense, by-the-book type of guy, and he insisted that she put absolutely no weight on her ankle for 90 days after her surgery. I think he must have intimidated her into full compliance - I can personally vouch that the bottom of her foot has never even brushed the ground during this time! Well this past Monday marked the 90th day, and she was cleared to start putting partial weight on it then.

I can't begin to explain how much we'd looked forward to this moment, especially because it signified a lot more than just 90 days after her last surgery, but *seven months* since her accident!

On Sunday night we were too excited to fall asleep, like two kids on Christmas eve. We stayed up watching trashy TV shows. At two minutes past midnight (thus officially following the doctor's orders for Monday), Mary Ann took her crutches and walked across the bedroom, gently putting her right ankle down with each step.

She said the ankle felt good. I was surprised at how naturally she walked. Her smile was radiant. We'll always treasure the small miracle of those first few steps, and the great work of the surgeon who put her mangled foot back together again.

This morning another small but significant step in our morning ritual: Mary Ann asked if *she* could bring up the coffee! For the first time since February, I stayed in bed while she went downstairs for the coffee. She could only manage one cup at a time, as she still needs to use one crutch to keep partial weight off her foot. But to see her enter the bedroom carrying that cup - wow...

Oct. 9 - More steps along the path

I recently had my monthly check-up with my Dana Farber cancer team. Overall the news was good. My liver functions are still off, but much better than last visit. As a reward, I even snuck a big glass of wine the other night at our neighbors' house. (But still don't tell the doctor.) The down side is that I'm having increased dryness and irritation in my eyes. The docs confirmed this was a common effect from GVH. Well as long as I can see my way down the ski slopes in another month or two, I'll be happy.

Anyway, sitting in the Dana Farber waiting room before my appointment, I looked around at all the different patients, each with their own personal cancer story. It was sort of a microcosm of our whole last year. There was one couple who was obviously there for the first time. Apparently the wife was going in for her blood lab, and the guy looked terrified. It reminded me that cancer is usually much harder on the spouse than on the patient - nobody has a clue until you've been there.

Dr. Soiffer, the head of our team, walked by. He's usually a jovial pleasant fellow who always says hello, but this time he had a dead serious look on his face as he strode past, went into an exam room where a family was waiting, and closed the door. (He never closes the door these days during my regular check-ups.) I assume he was having "the conversation" with them, something else that you can never grasp unless you've lived it.

I noticed another guy in the waiting area looking particularly weak and emaciated. I could barely see his dark sunken eyes over his face mask. He was wearing rubber gloves, his hands trembling. I remembered what it was like during my visits last winter, when I was all masked and gloved, shaking, too weak to stand for more than 30 seconds. I wondered if this guy would make it back like I did.

And then there was one of the "veterans" nearby, holding a cup of Dunkin Donuts coffee and wearing his Red Sox cap, as so many patients seem to do. A friendly, talkative guy with a great Boston accent. We started chatting about the Sox pitching staff, the playoffs - all the usual Boston stuff. It was so typical of the warmth and comradery in that cancer waiting room. Go check it out sometime if you want to see the human spirit at its best.

Speaking of the human spirit, I want to share one more amazing thing that happened to me recently. In the condominium community where we live, I've been working for the past few years on cutting a trail alongside our little pond. For obvious reasons, I haven't been able to work on it much during the past year and a half. But a few neighbors kept it going, and recently they got it finished. A few days ago, they called me down to the path to show me a surprise. They'd made a sign modeled after the National Forest trail signs, and installed it just inside the entrance to the path. It read "Peter's Path."

I was totally surprised and deeply touched. Apparently the idea for this sign began last fall, when they weren't sure whether I was going to make it. Of course, I kidded the guys that I'd fooled them by coming back to enjoy my "memorial" path while I'm still around! We had a few laughs over that. My dream now is that Mary Ann will soon be well enough to walk down that path with me.

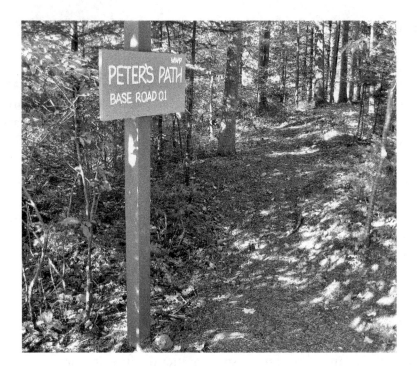

Oct 26 - The path (continued)

Not a lot of medical updates here the last couple weeks because Mary Ann and I have been consumed by more normal stuff like errands and community activities and zipping all over the US with work travel. This all probably sounds mundane and insignificant, which is exactly the point. It's been great to get a taste of our old, busy lives back.

And best of all, following from the previous post, this afternoon we took that first walk together down Peter's Path.

Nov. 1, 2009 – The start of Year Two

When you go through an experience like this, you tend to quantify the passage of time, paying special attention to major anniversaries and milestones. Remember, for example, how significant that 100-day post-transplant milestone once seemed?

These milestones give you goals to strive for. Even if they're just arbitrary dates, they help focus your energy, maybe even help keep you sane. And once they're past, they give you benchmarks to look back upon and mark how far you've come.

Well yesterday was a huge milestone - the one year anniversary of my transplant. I can't begin to describe even a tiny fraction of all my thoughts and feelings as I passed into Year Two. So guess what - I won't even try.

Nov. 24 - Childhood all over again

Today I had to go back down to Dana Farber again for another purpose: to receive my childhood immunization shots. That's right - I had to get those same shots fifty or so years after the first time around! This is because my immune system is just starting to rebuild itself all over again. It's a continuation of the process I wrote about when I had my transplant, the way they called it my "birthday." Well now I'm in my childhood, and it's time to get my shots.

This of course prompted lots of jokes from Mary Ann as I headed out: "Are you gonna cry? Do you think they'll give you a lollipop?" and so on.

My appointment went fine, and it was sort of fun kidding with the nurse as she gave me the shots. (And no, I didn't cry - no lollipop, either!) But it was what took place *before* my appointment that I'd like to tell you about. Several things happened in close proximity to each other. Nothing major - just a confluence of simple, little everyday occurrences. But taken together, they made me scratch my head and wonder about human nature. I think you'll see what I mean.

On the way to the hospital, the heavy city traffic was crawling slowly through the congested area. As I approached an intersection, the light was green, but the traffic was all clogged ahead. So I didn't go through, because I'd only go a few feet and end up blocking the intersection. Well you should have seen the guy behind me, blowing his horn, gesturing wildly, and generally going nuts for me to move ahead - which would only have netted him a grand total of about two car lengths.

I got into the elevator coming up from the parking garage. The elevator door was starting to close when a woman came into the lobby frantically shrieking to hold the door open. We couldn't stop it in time, and the door closed without her. I looked over at the other guy in the elevator, we each smiled and just shook our heads - how that woman practically blew a gasket over having to wait maybe another thirty seconds to catch the next elevator up.

In the lobby I checked my emails. I found myself in the crossfires of two separate "Reply All" squabbles among neighbors, each filled with harsh tone and lots of expletives flying back and forth. People going absolutely ballistic. The two issues? One involved a single tree a guy cut down to improve his (and everyone's) view; the other was about a proposed schedule change with the shuttle service that goes around our resort. Real earth-shattering stuff, eh? It makes you wonder how people can get so worked up about relatively minor things.

Anyway, before my appointment for the shots, I had to go for a bone density test at another building down the street. On my way back to Dana Farber, I passed by the entrance to Children's Hospital. I had some time to kill, and I remembered from my training presentations there over the years that they have an outstanding Au Bon Pain in the lobby - absolutely killer Asiago cheese bagels. (This is the kind of stuff I remember.) So I went in for a quick bite.

Well the bagel was delicious, but I soon forgot all about it as I watched the scene in the Children's Hospital lobby: Little kids everywhere, many in braces or wheelchairs, many hooked to tubes, many with bald heads. And they were all so wide-eyed and innocent and sweet - none looked scared. The lobby is full of bright colors and all sorts of displays and games. They have this amazing Rube Goldberg type contraption with rolling balls and clanging bells, and I just stood there mesmerized watching it with a gaggle of wide-eyed kids.

As I watched the scene all around, it suddenly dawned on me what my next appointment was: getting my own "childhood" immunization shots. In other words, getting a second crack at life after a pretty good 56 years the first time around. And it hit me hard when I realized how many of those sweet innocent kids in the lobby might never even get the chance to... well, you know what I mean.

So if you're ever feeling sorry for yourself, or stressed about some insignificant thing, go hang out in the Children's Hospital lobby for a while. It'll touch your heart, and realign your priorities.

Happy Thanksgiving.

Dec. 3, 2009 - Back at line-up

Over the weekend, I returned to a beloved and familiar place for the first time in 20 months: the morning "line-up" of ski instructors waiting for our lessons. You feel a special warmth and camaraderie out there with the gang. Maybe it's because we're in a beautiful place doing something we love, and helping others in the process. It was a joy to be back...

Notes from the present day

A few quick updates here as we moved into my Year Two. Yes, that ski season got off to a great start, and continued all winter. Although far from my peak, I held up OK. And every time I looked out at that amazing view, I felt awe and gratitude.

Health wise, everything was moving along for both of us. I kept feeling stronger, and Mary Ann's ankle was continuing to heal well. Her knee doctor was waiting for that leg to get strong enough to become the dominant one. Then he'd do the surgery on her other knee. It was nice to be able to plan ahead strategically.

Unfortunately, the problems continued at the real estate office. The new development was long gone, leaving a lot of bad vibes and ill will in its wake. The condo resale volume was slow, as you'd expect with the miserable economy, and eventually Mary Ann was laid off there as well.

She didn't spend much time wallowing around. She immediately got to work hustling up a new business venture. She started a little concierge service for resort visitors. I pitched in as much as I could. It was sort of fun, but not very lucrative. Mary Ann also started sending out feelers to contacts in the broadcasting industry.

My corporate training volume was slowly coming back, plus I was bringing in a few extra bucks with my ski instructing. Even so, it was a bit of a jolt when I realized that the primary breadwinner role had shifted onto my shoulders!

And then, when the specter of health insurance starting rearing its ugly head, our life really fell into panic mode again.

More on that later, but now I'd like to go back to the blog briefly and share a post from this point in the chronology. It doesn't need much context from me – I think it speaks for itself.

Jan. 26, 2010 - Haiti and human nature

In the past couple weeks, we've watched a lot of the stories about the earthquake in Haiti. Most of the sights have been horrifying and sad.

But disasters often seem to bring out the best in the human spirit. It's been great to see how many people - government leaders, doctors, and private citizens - have all pitched in to help in their own way. Some doctors we know are down there right now, volunteering their help. The other day I was at the check-out counter at a store and watched a little kid read the sign on a collection jar for Haiti earthquake relief, reach into his pocket, and drop some change into the slot.

Especially in these polarized times, it's been encouraging to see people of different political views and religions all unified in their goodwill toward the Haitians. Bush and Clinton working together, so many different nations and churches offering aid, and so on.

Sort of reminds me of the way so many different people from all backgrounds and religions and political views have all pitched in to help Mary Ann and me over the past couple years. With all our medical problems, we've been blessed to see human nature at its best.

Unfortunately, however, there always seem to be a few exceptions - people who respond to disasters and others' suffering in the most repugnant way. For example, several media pundits have actually criticized President Obama for responding to the earthquake so decisively, saying he only did so because he's a "black helping other blacks." One popular media figure blamed the Haitians for their own suffering, saying it was God's will to punish them for their religious practices. Reminds me of the nut cases who show up at the funerals of soldiers who die in Iraq & Afghanistan, saying they "deserved to die" because of the US policy toward gays. Hard to believe humans can act like this.

Bringing it back to our situation, Mary Ann confided something to me the other day that I never knew: She said that a couple people at her former real estate job had told her that I *deserved my cancer* because I'm a Jew who had not "accepted Christ." Wow, can you believe anybody would say that? To tell the truth, I've always admired Jesus and "accepted" his inspiring lessons about compassion and tolerance – qualities many of these folks sure don't seem to practice. It just makes me shake my head and wonder – what's happened to the fundamental spirit of human decency that I thought was supposed to underlie all religions?

Fortunately, this type of ignorance has been only a tiny fraction of our experience, and the vast majority of people have been wonderful. Let's do everything we can to keep it that way.

Notes from the present day

As I said above, I think I'll let the previous post speak for itself. It speaks volumes...

Anyway, we kept scraping along during that winter. Mary Ann had her knee surgery in February, which went well. Even though she was back on crutches for a while, she recovered fast, and we felt optimistic (at least with our health).

My revenue picked up enough to the point where I told Social Security they could take me off my disability. For the most part that felt great – but it was also a bit scary.

Speaking of scary, let's go back to the blog for a while. The first post is another type of health scare, but then everything takes an upward turn from there.

March 6, 2010 - A scare

This past week Mary Ann came with me on my trip to the Boston area. I had several medical appointments and a business writing workshop to lead. We decided it would be easier for her to hang out at my hotel, order room service, etc. rather than be home alone struggling to carry things up & down the stairs. It was delightful traveling with her.

My work went great. Though my eyes were really bothering me, I felt the old magic being back on top of my game running the workshop.

My cancer appointment also resulted in some good news - my red blood counts have climbed back into the normal range! Red blood cells are the ones that carry oxygen through the body. For someone as physically active as me, you can imagine how exciting this was. As it soon turned out, however, a bit on the ironic side.

On the ride back up to NH, I started feeling a tightness in my chest and a pressing pain each time I inhaled. I just couldn't seem to get a deep breath. When we stopped for gas, I went to the trunk and quietly took an aspirin out of my suitcase.

As we continued north, I told Mary Ann that I wasn't feeling so great, but kept it pretty low-key. Secretly, however, I was thinking ahead about each upcoming exit, trying to anticipate where the hospitals were just in case.

With the help of U2 booming through the car stereo, we made it home OK and soon fell asleep. At about 2:00 am, I awoke to go to the bathroom. As soon as I stood up, I felt a sharp constriction in my chest. I stayed awake in bed for a while, trying to recover my breath. But the weight on my chest seemed to get heavier, and my mind kept racing. I thought of the many people I've known who've had heart attacks, including Mary Ann's dad and my own father, who died suddenly from a heart problem less than 11 months ago. For one of the very few times during this whole journey, I felt fear.

Like many guys, I was tempted to just lie in bed stoically, to tough it out, to wait till morning, to spare Mary Ann from worry or inconvenience. But a huge lesson we've learned from this adventure is that an attitude of stoic, macho denial is really stupid - and the exact *opposite* of being considerate to the other person.

So I woke up Mary Ann and told her I think we needed to go to the hospital. She was up and dressed in world record time, though surprisingly calm (at least on the outside). The 2:30 am drive through the dark NH night felt surprisingly peaceful, and familiar too.

And so was the Littleton Hospital Emergency Room. As usual, the staff there were great getting me all checked in, hooked up to all sorts of tubes and electrodes and monitors. The front wall of my room was all glass, and Mary Ann and I were stunned looking around and realizing how many of the different ER rooms we'd patronized before: Over there was the room where she was treated for her near-fatal ear infection. Next to it was where they plucked & vacuumed the glass shards out of me after my moose collision. Nearby was the room where they treated my stomach infection soon after my transplant. Across the way we saw where they wheeled her in last February with her shattered ankle (which sent a shudder through both of us). And down the hall was the room where I took her a few weeks later as she writhed in pain.

The ER team started running a whole bunch of tests on me: EKG, CT scan, ultrasound, etc. And they also gave me a succession of different drugs: Nitro-glycerin, morphine, anti-inflammatories, etc., monitoring the results from each. I was impressed how methodically they proceeded to rule things out and isolate exactly what was going on. I was also impressed with the way the ER doc called in his colleague to help make sure he got the assessment right - great humility and teamwork - and all this at 4:00 am!

Bottom line was that I did *not* have a heart attack. In fact, their tests assured me that most of my heart functions were strong. Instead, my problem was a severe, GVH-induced inflammation of the heart lining called pericarditis. Though I felt many of the same symptoms of a heart attack, this was much less dangerous.

The short-term outlook: No heavy exertion, lots of anti-inflammatories, a few more tests this week to make sure of the diagnosis, and no skiing for at least a few days.

So here we sit on the bed, sipping our coffee, each of us typing away on our laptops, the beautiful ski trails out the window beckoning but off limits to us both.

March 30 - Two milestones on the road back

Milestones come in all different sizes, shapes, and forms. Here are a couple recent ones for us, totally different in scope but both encouraging steps forward.

1) Rarely do you feel a tangible impact from something in Washington, but with the passage of the Affordable Care Act, our world changed a bit. I've been fortunate to have had good health coverage so far, but when Mary Ann was terminated from her real estate job, we lost that sense of security. COBRA extended my coverage temporarily, but the clock was ticking down. When my COBRA expired, I would have been unable to get health care coverage ever again due to my pre-existing condition. God knows how we would have managed. Well those days are over, and this opens up a whole new world of security and opportunity for us. Our deepest thanks to the leadership and guts of President Obama.

2) I mentioned a few posts ago that Mary Ann had been getting encouraging job inquiries. Well much has happened since then. Guess what? Right now she's upstairs in her home office, hard at work on the second day of her new job! She's the Executive Director for North American Business Development (or some fancy title like that) for a company that makes audio equipment for the broadcast industry. Ever since her hiring was announced in a press release, phone calls and emails have been pouring in from former colleagues (and even competitors) around the world, congratulating her and welcoming her back to the industry. I've never seen her so energized.

April 8 - We learned who my donor is!

The most amazing thing happened yesterday. I got a letter from the Dana Farber Cancer Institute, and they finally identified the person who donated his stem cells to me - the person who helped save my life.

For over a year-and-a-half, ever since we got the thrilling news that they found a perfect match for me, this donor was an anonymous, faceless angel out there somewhere - we always wondered who & where - until yesterday.

When I opened that envelope and this person suddenly took on a specific identity, all sorts of emotions welled up inside of me. I showed it to Mary Ann, and we both sat there stunned, deeply moved.

Anyway, the guy's name is Eric, he's 23, a recent grad from Syracuse. As soon as I finish this entry, I'm going to write to him. Usually the words flow easily for me, but I have no idea how in the world I can properly express our gratitude.

April 29, 2010 - "He broke up with me"

Mary Ann and I have had several appointments with our various doctors all bunched together over the last few days. I noticed they all had a common theme.

My meeting at Dana Farber showed mostly good blood readings, though my red blood counts have once again dipped back below the normal range. If you know me, you know I was quietly pissed on the inside. But Dr. Soiffer wasn't concerned, and he even lowered my immune-suppressant drug by a half MG per day, which might seem like a tiny step but is actually a giant leap. And one more small marker of progress: He scheduled my next appointment for two-and-a-half months later - the longest interval yet! You get so used to the rhythm of regular monthly appointments, and when they extend them out longer, at first it feels a bit unsettling, then thrilling.

Mary Ann met with her knee doctor recently. He was so impressed with her progress that he didn't even schedule a follow-up visit. As happy as she was to hear his assessment, she said it felt odd not to have another appointment on the books.

And then came her appointment with Dr. Trauma the other day. He checked out her ankle thoroughly, and said it had healed as well as possible. He said she could do whatever she could tolerate on it - hike, bike, jog, even jump! That was so exciting to hear!

Then he discharged her. It would be up to another doctor eventually to determine her degree of permanent impairment, but Trauma's work was done.

What an amazing bit of news. And what a jolt. We've grown to look forward to our visits there, to enjoy the familiar faces, the playful banter, the mayhem and zany cast of characters at that inner-city hospital. We've grown accustomed to the automatic scheduling of the next visit, to the secure feeling that she was constantly in the capable hands of Dr. T, the man who rescued her ankle from the butchery of last winter and spring.

But suddenly we were on our own.

As we made our way out through the lobby, all sorts of emotions were stirring: relief, joy, even a touch of sadness. Suddenly Mary Ann put on a long face, her lip quivered, and in mock despair she blurted out, "He broke up with me." God I love how funny she is! We both laughed as we traded the usual break-up lines: ("he's just not that into you anymore... he wants to see other people... he's not ready for commitment," etc.) Typical of us, the way we try to find humor in almost everything.

But I felt something else welling up in me - a surprising feeling of release. This marked the end of a 14 month nightmare, a nightmare that started with Mary Ann's shattered ankle bones, but eventually enveloped our lives in more ways than you can imagine. Though my tear ducts aren't working these days, I could sure feel them wanting to.

Notes from the present day

The walk out of the hospital that day was a huge turning point. It felt as if we'd made it over the hump. Our medical issues certainly didn't disappear, but they receded enough so we could get back to living our lives.

I stopped writing in my blog. Several readers said they missed my posts, even worried when so much time went by. I knew I'd get around to a final post eventually – I was just waiting for a theme to tie it all together...

During a warm night that summer, Mary Ann and I had just come out of a movie at the little theater in Bethlehem. We were standing in line at the ice cream shop next door, when behind us I noticed Dr. Diener. You might remember Dr. Diener as the first oncologist I saw when this whole journey began. He was the one who showed so much compassion as he broke the news that I had cancer. I'll never forget his kind manner as he guided us through that frightening time.

Anyway, as I paid for our ice cream cones, I gave the clerk a few extra dollars and told her to pay for the guy in line behind us. Dr. Diener made the obligatory "You don't have to do that" protest, but I wouldn't hear of it. As I said to him, "Doc, a lousy ice cream cone? Come on, that's the least I can do." What an understatement that was.

That little ice-cream encounter gave me the topic for my final blog post. Yes, it was time to say thank you. But I wanted to do it in a more original way than one of those trite "I-just-want-to-thank..." Academy Award speeches. I got to thinking about a crazy musical escapade Mary Ann and I had gone on the year before, and suddenly it all came together. I had the idea for my final post. And I'd like to take you back there now.

August, 2010 – My final post: Inspiration from Leonard Cohen

Hello again. Welcome back! I'm not sure how many people are still with me, especially after I've let so much time pass between posts. But even if nobody's reading, this last entry is something *I* really want to do. Here goes.

Soon after we started making our numerous drives down to Boston for medical appointments, I noticed that Mary Ann loved to play (and sing along to) Leonard Cohen CD's. Now I never thought that much of Leonard Cohen – I knew he wrote a few good songs, and like everyone from my era of course I remembered that sleepy one about Suzanne taking you down to the river. But I always wrote him off as a washed-up relic from the 60's, a dreary-voiced troubadour of disillusionment and depression.

I enjoyed teasing Mary Ann about her Leonard Cohen obsession. At the same time, I got a kick out of her fascination with his songs, especially his quirky lyrics.

So way back last May, I decided to surprise her by getting us tickets to Leonard Cohen's show in Boston. We'd been virtual shut-ins for almost a year, but I figured we were getting well enough (barely) to step out again. I was recovered just enough from my transplant to go out in public again, albeit with a mask on and a bottle of hand sanitizer in my pocket. And Mary Ann was about eight weeks past her second surgery, limping gingerly with a brace on her leg, her doctor having given her clearance to start walking again. (Mistakenly, as it turned out.)

We made our way down to Boston and somehow hobbled our way into the Citi Center. We must have been quite a pathetic sight, me with my mask and peach fuzzy head, and Mary Ann with her severe, distorted limp. But it felt exciting to be back out among a big crowd for a night on the town. As we often say to make fun of our remote mountain existence, "We don't get out much."

The lights went down, the band came out, and then out walked this ancient looking guy with a rumpled grey suit and top-hat. The crowd roared. It was Leonard. They started right into "Dance Me to the End of Love." I'd always thought that was a Madeline Peyroux song – I had no idea that Leonard Cohen had written and recorded it years before. The band was incredible, with some of the best musicians I've ever heard. Within a few bars, I was hooked. And Leonard himself was mesmerizing, this wrinkled old man, often dropping onto one knee as he cupped the mike to his mouth, his voice as dreary and off-key as ever.

Even though the Citi Center is huge, with about 4,000 seats, the stage had sort of a dark, intimate feeling. Deep blue light, like a smoky jazz club. Perfect.

As the show went on, I kept glancing at Mary Ann - she was beaming, sometimes even singing along. After all that she'd been through with my year of cancer and her three months of ankle pain... well you can see why it felt so wonderful to be enjoying such a night out. And I have to admit, I was loving the show myself more than I expected - along with the smug satisfaction of knowing that I'd nailed it with this surprise gift to my wife.

Just before intermission, they played a song I later learned was called "Anthem." I wasn't familiar with it, but it grabbed me right away with its beautiful, almost spiritual sound. At first the lyrics seemed to echo a familiar Leonard Cohen theme, lamenting all the disappointments and imperfections in the world. But at the end of the chorus, he dropped in a line that stunned me, and has resonated with me ever since:

> *Ring the bells that still can ring*
> *Forget your perfect offering*
> *There's a crack, a crack in everything*
> *That's how the light gets in*

Each time they played this verse, when they got to that last line the lights came up, suddenly washing the stage with a yellow glow. It was awesome...

...And in the fifteen months since that show, not a day has passed when I haven't thought of that line, *"That's how the light gets in."*

Yes, despite all the difficulties (or maybe I should say "cracks") in our life the last two-and-a half years, we've been blessed by countless rays of light shining through the darkness.

One way the light has touched us has been through the amazing gestures of support, generosity, and love we've received from others. I'll never be able to cite them all, but a few examples come to mind:

When I was in the hospital, my long-time friend Johnny I bringing in a beautiful framed photo he took of the Presidential Mountains to remind me of home - and maybe give me a little incentive to get back there.

My brothers and sisters-in-law delivering a copy of Will Ferrell's "Talladega Nights" to keep my spirits up in the hospital.

Every visitor who made the effort to find their way to my sealed off hospital ward, and put on a mask and gloves and sanitizer - each one a ray of light shining into my little room.

Mary Ann's sister flying up from Maryland to spend several days frantically scrubbing every inch of our house spotless prior to my hospital release.

When I was quarantined at home, unable to go out, barely able to walk, my ski instructor buddies calling me on their cell phone from the ski hill, telling me to grab the binoculars and look out the window, where I could see them all waving from the side of the ski trail.

Or throwing snowballs against my window one below-zero afternoon to get my attention, where I looked out and saw them making snow angels in our yard.

Johnny G organizing a quiet fundraiser, completely unknown to me, and then driving three hours up to NH one morning to surprise us with a check.

A whole group of work colleagues spending months secretly making a mobile of 1,000 origami cranes, a Japanese tradition to help people recover from illness. I guess it worked.

Daniel and Jim and a few other neighbors deciding to name a path after me, secretly building and installing a sign modeled after the National Forest trail signs in the nearby White Mountains.

When Mary Ann was unable to walk and I could barely leave the house, her Book Club colleagues making out a schedule to cook us dinners, and then every single member following through right on schedule, delivering a hot steaming meal to our door at the appointed time.

Every time the power went out, our neighbors Curt & Margaret calling within minutes, offering to share their generator-powered home with us.

Or Peg & Albert bringing over their plastic shower chair every time Mary Ann had another surgery.

My eighty-year-old mother moving in with us, cooking and cleaning, playing jigsaw puzzles and Scrabble, and even shoveling the snow off our deck when we couldn't.

From our community, countless drop-by visits, offers of rides, shopping, errands, meals cooked & delivered, flowers, and little gifts.

From near and far, countless calls, cards, emails, and touching comments on this blog.

And so much more. Every gesture, no matter how small, a bright ray of light. The best of human nature shining through.

Leonard Cohen's words have given us a vehicle to appreciate another source of light during our journey. There's been a lot of noise about our health care system in the last couple years, and it's been interesting to go through this whole experience against that backdrop. Whatever your political views, I think everyone can agree that the health care system can be a chaotic, confusing, often frustrating quagmire. We've sure struggled to navigate our way through it. But through the many "cracks" in that mess, we've been warmed by so many shining rays of light from the many wonderful health care providers who have helped us along the way.

For example, the Littleton Hospital ER team and ear doc, who calmly went right to work when I rushed Mary Ann in with blood streaming out of her ear, in agonizing pain, her infection starting to enter her brain. Though to them it was probably just another day's work, they saved my wife's life.

The grace and kind manner of Dr. Diener, our local oncologist who first broke the news that I had cancer – the calm, compassionate way he took the time to explain things, answer questions, acknowledge my uncertainty and fears. Never the least bit in a rush.

And the rest of Diener's oncology staff, who warmly welcomed me as the "newbie" into the surprisingly upbeat chemotherapy ward during that first scary summer.

The pleasant guy who ran the radiation room at Brigham & Women's Hospital, who over four days calmly administered enough radiation through that monstrous machine on the ceiling to zap most of my blood cells and come close to killing the rest of me. I never caught his name, but I'll always remember how he put me at ease, and let me choose the music during my treatments.

The phlebotomy staff at Dana Farber, most of whom seemed to be from the Caribbean for some reason, always smiling at my jokes about how many vials of blood they're taking from me, but always focused to get that stick in painlessly the first time every time. Real pros.

The nurses' assistants and maids in the hospital cancer ward, surrounded by so much sickness, performing so many menial and unpleasant tasks taking care of us... but always ready to greet you with a smile, a ray of light shining in every time I heard that double air-lock door creak open.

And the nurses themselves, each with their own personality and style, all incredibly competent, caring, and professional. What a noble profession.

My head nurse Nejor, telling me tales of growing up in East Africa dreaming of coming to the States one day, calmly administering the stem cells that trickled through my bloodstream into my bone marrow and gave me new life. What an inspiring story.

The ER staff at Littleton Hospital (again), so calm and professional when I stumbled in there with my stomach infection eating away at my insides, weaker and sicker than I've ever been, wondering if this might be it. And the woman at the registration desk who checked me in, looked me deep in the eyes and said "I'll be praying for you" as they wheeled me into the ER – I noticed a tear in her eye. The light really shines through when you see that type of compassion from somebody "just doing their job."

Even some folks who were not direct care providers, but important parts of the system, were surprising rays of light while just doing their jobs: Pat, the workers comp administrator at our local resort, who steadfastly managed Mary Ann's case amidst a sea of hassles and resistance from her real estate managers; the folks from Social Security, who smoothly and compassionately helped me file a disability claim when I was unable to work for over a year; even several people we dealt with from the dreaded insurance companies who were warm, efficient, and caring. Bright rays of light all.

Unfortunately, Mary Ann had some health providers from whom we couldn't find much light, especially early in her broken ankle nightmare. But in a way, this only made us appreciate all the more the good ones we eventually encountered along the way. For example:

The foot doc at NE Baptist - an orthopedic hospital so renowned that they treat Boston pro athletes - who had the bluntness to tell us that the previous shoddy work on her ankle "pissed him off," the humility to say that even he and his colleagues were not up to fixing it, and the graciousness to recommend someone at a competing hospital as the only one in the region capable of repairing her damage. A special type of light shining in during a time of frustration and uncertainty.

And that brings us to Dr. Trauma, the surgeon who took on the challenge of repairing Mary Ann's ankle, fixing the damage not just from her fall but from two ineffective surgeries and shoddy follow-up care. So focused, some might even say intimidating, that during our first few meetings he'd stride in without saying hello, proceed right to the x-ray display, and start dictating what he saw and what he was going to do. We'd occasionally overhear him in the hall telling his nurse that he would no longer treat certain patients who were "non-cooperative." He'd lecture us that his restrictions were "non-negotiable." We joked that this intimidating manner was just an act to get our attention, and in fact we found it quite endearing. Because underneath we saw a man of incredible focus, preparation, and yes, even warmth. One time as we were leaving an appointment, he could tell that Mary Ann was feeling a bit worried about her future. Dr. T looked in her eyes, gave an encouraging smile, reached out and hugged her. The reassuring light of competence, confidence, and compassion shining through.

And speaking of competence, of course there's Dr. Soiffer, my head cancer doc at Dana Farber - one of the brightest lights of all. So down-to-earth, so human, so comfortable with the huge responsibilities in his hands. I'll never forget the way he calmly and bluntly outlined the grim statistics of my survival chances, and then patted me on the shoulder and said 'You'll do fine." Or when I was in the hospital, the time he said I was doing so well that I was "boring." Just recently during one of my regular visits, he suddenly left the exam room – at first I wondered if he'd been paged for a medical emergency, but then he rushed back in and excitedly updated me on the winning goal from the US World Cup soccer game. This from the man who led the team that saved my life.

I've really struggled to find an appropriate way to say thanks and give something back to the great staff at Dana Farber. Sure, I send them a little check every so often for their fund-raising drives. I've signed up for every study and clinical trial they've asked me to join, hoping in some small way to contribute to their body of research. I've offered to be a mentor or resource to other cancer & transplant patients. I've worked to promote bone marrow registration drives to help add to the pool of prospective donors. And one of these days, I'll try to find the words to express my thanks to Dr. Soiffer.

Say what you will about our health care system, but don't forget to appreciate all the wonderful people who work in it, shining rays of light to those in need.

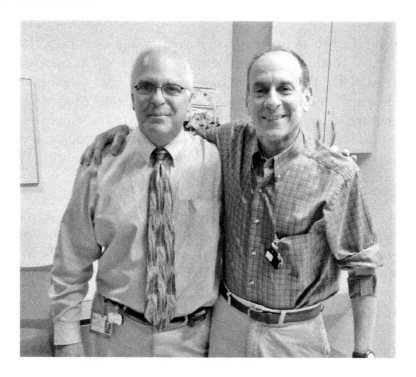

The light can shine through the cracks even in times of great pain. One of the most remarkable (and literal) examples of this occurred last April, the morning after my father Bob suddenly died. Read that entry from April 21 of 2009. I wrote it at the crack of dawn, on a raw, drizzly April morning, snow still on the ski trails across the street, and the sky cold grey. I was still in shock, stunned, it all had happened so suddenly the night before. The first morning in 55 years that I awoke without a father. I tried to find solace that he died quickly, without suffering, at least I hoped so. I wondered if he had felt as relieved and uplifted as I did from my visit just four days before. As was I finishing up that post, a rainbow suddenly appeared for a few seconds - a rarity that time of year. In those fleeting seconds that I gazed out at the rainbow, with rays of sunlight somehow poking through the grey clouds, I knew that my father was at peace and everything was all right. It felt warm and comforting.

Bringing this all back to the present day, Mary Ann is out in Nebraska, helping her parents bring home a new puppy from a breeder several hours away. Their beloved dog Sarah died of old age a couple months ago, leaving a void in their lives. Mary Ann made the effort to take a 24-hour round trip out there because she wanted to help them restore some light back into their lives. If you've ever had a pet, you know what I mean.

When she was home last weekend, we decided we were ready to try climbing a 4,000 footer. That's the benchmark for the taller peaks around here, the elevation where the footing gets steep and rough, and you start to reach the spectacular area above timberline. We hadn't done a 4,000 footer together in three years. So we trudged up Mt. Jackson, a peak that looks down on our resort valley. We went slowly, carefully, each of us laboring far more than we used to. But we made it!

A little over a year after Dr. T rebuilt Mary Ann's mangled ankle, twenty-two months after I received the transplant of new life, you could hear the bells ringing, and see the light shining, as we celebrated on the peak.

And that brings me to the greatest light of all through this long journey. I hope I've been able to show it, so I won't spend much time saying it. But with all the hardships and struggles we've faced the last few years - all the "cracks" in our life if you will - the light that has streamed through most brightly and steadily of all to me has been the unwavering beacon of love from my amazing wife Mary Ann. I only hope I've been able to shine a little light of my own back her way – she sure deserves it, and so much more.

My thanks to all who have helped us through this adventure. My thanks to Leonard Cohen, who inspired us to find beauty and optimism amid life's challenges. And my thanks to you for sticking with me through this blog. Please stay in touch, take care of each other, and be well.

Notes from the present day

And that was it. My blog was done. (Or so I thought, as you'll soon see.) And it remained "done" for well over a year.

On Halloween night, October 31, 2010, I completed Year Two and passed into Year Three. Soon afterward I got my two-year immunization shots. (Still no lollipop!)

My health remained steady throughout Year Three, with mostly encouraging reports from my continued visits down to Dana Farber. Same symptoms, but not too bad.

Speaking of Dana Farber, they opened a sparkling new building. Much more spacious and modern, but somehow I missed the character of the old place.

The economy was climbing back from the great recession - maybe more slowly than we'd like, and possibly never to the level it was before, but clearly on the upswing. Come to think of it, that was a good description of my health.

Mary Ann was back in the groove with her work. Sometimes I overheard her on the phone with her broadcasting clients, and she sure had that zest and magic back in her voice.

Her ankle and knee improved overall, though with some lingering pain, especially when hiking downhill. We kept hiking that summer and fall, eventually reaching another milestone: the summit of Mt Lafayette, one of the few 5,000-footers in New Hampshire. It was amazing to be back up in the world above timberline with my wife again. And that winter, for the first time in *three years*, we shared some great skiing together.

Not everything was good news. As Mary Ann and I discovered so dramatically when she slipped on that icy path, your entire life can change in a split second. Well the same thing happened with my mother Nancy. She took a bad fall on some outdoor steps, shattering her leg and elbow.

We rushed down to visit her in the hospital. I'll never forget walking into her room. Foggy and barely coherent from painkillers, she was all wrapped in casts and bandages, tubes in her nose, IV hooked up to her arm, red blotches and bruises all over - she was a mess. For the first time in my life, I thought she looked old. For the first time in my life, I thought of her mortality.

The nurses had brought in a tray with some soup, but lying back in the bed, with one arm wrapped in bandages and the other tangled in IV tubes, Nancy couldn't manage to eat it. So I grabbed the spoon, leaned over, and fed her some soup. You can imagine all the thoughts and feelings I had about that - a whole world of symbolism there.

Anyway, she recovered well at the hospital and soon went into a long stay at a rehab facility. I'll hold off telling you the rest of the story here, because guess what? I ended up writing another blog post! I called it my Epilogue. It'll fill you in on the rest of Nancy's story, as well as the twists and turns of our own journey.

It will take our story through Year Three and into Year Four. And as you'll see, it also propelled me forward in ways far more meaningful than year count.

THE CLIMB OUT

That Epilogue turned out to be the last of my blog entries. Yes, really, it did. So let's go back to December of 2011, and a life-changing trip. Afterwards, I'll bring the rest of this narrative back to the present-day perspective with which it began.

Part 7

REFLECTIONS FROM ISRAEL

December, 2011 – Epilogue: A trip to Israel

Hello again! Well it's been sixteen months since my so-called "final" blog post. During that time many people have asked me to keep my blog going (which I find very flattering). We've also had some new twists in this journey that could have made for interesting entries. However, I really meant it last August when I said that was the end - probably as an attempt to impose some closure on this whole thing and move on. And to tell the truth, I thought that last entry was a pretty good way to close.

So I really haven't had any temptations to write more. That is, until now.

I'm typing this in a hotel in Tel Aviv, Israel. Sitting at a computer in the concierge lounge. Looking out over the Mediterranean, with the sunset glowing orange way out on the horizon. Feeling the sand that's still between my toes from our walk along the beach a while ago. Reflecting on what has been an amazing day. No, "amazing" isn't quite the right word - maybe moving or inspiring would be more accurate. In any case, it's been a day that, among many other things, gave me the spark to take a stab at writing this epilogue to my cancer blog. You'll see why.

So what's gone on in the past year? Well I certainly don't want to overwhelm you with a complete chronology, but let me share a few random highlights that pop into my mind. I'd like to start with a story about my mother Nancy. You might have heard that last October she had a terrible fall with a broken leg and arm.

Nancy ended up spending over two months recovering in a "rehab" institution. I put "rehab" in quotes because we all know what that place must have felt like. All the residents were old, many were suffering from dementia, and some would probably never leave there alive. You can imagine how depressing it must have been to be confined there for so long. But my mother had great support from friends and family, and her care was good. She also put a lot of effort into her physical therapy exercises. As a result, she made a remarkable recovery. And she demonstrated a valuable lesson for recoveries of all kinds: Sometimes you have to put some work into getting better.

Nancy's release day was very special. As Mary Ann and I picked her up to take her home, it was touching to see all the warm goodbyes from the staff - I'm sure they don't always get to see such a successful departure. But I sensed there was something deeper going on, and I think I know why. Occasionally during my visits, I overheard other patients being grouchy and demanding toward the staff, but I noticed that Nancy treated them with courtesy and gratitude. Most were immigrants from the Caribbean and Africa, doing menial tasks like emptying bedpans and taking patients to the bathroom. Tough work. I'm sure paid very low wages. As they said goodbye to Nancy, you could tell that their good wishes were heartfelt. I flashed back to my own departure after my long transplant confinement – very similar, with warm goodbyes and hugs from the staff, most of whom were also immigrants. I'd like to think I learned a thing or two about treating others from my mother.

So we walked Nancy down the hall toward the exit, pressed the button on the automated double doors, and burst outside into the cold, refreshing air. She hadn't been outside for over two months. Again, I flashed back to my own release day three years earlier. After you've been confined for so long, especially in a large institutional place, there's just something magical about that first breath of real outdoor air.

We drove my mother home, stocked her refrigerator with food, and got her settled into her apartment. The most important task of all? Connecting her computer and getting her TV hooked up with the clicker in easy reach. Sounds sort of tongue-in-cheek trivial, but I'm being totally serious. There's no more potent medicine than returning to the familiar comforts of home. Also, things like phones, clickers, and computers might seem like impersonal gadgets, but they serve a powerful purpose: keeping someone - especially a widow in her eighties – connected to the world. It felt nice to remember all that when turning the tables and becoming a caregiver for someone else.

Speaking of which, in typical Nancy fashion, she'd made a hair appointment for that very afternoon. After two months in a drab, institutional rehab facility, I'm sure you can see why it was so important for her to get her hair done. Soon after we got her settled at home, it was time for her appointment. It was at a salon a couple blocks from her apartment, normally about a two minute walk. But unfortunately it had started snowing and blowing like crazy. Any reasonable person would stay indoors in those conditions, not to mention an 82 year old woman on a cane recovering from a shattered leg and arm.

But I knew something about that little hair appointment, and I said let's go. Nancy didn't hesitate. She grabbed my arm with one hand and leaned gingerly on her cane with the other, and we shuffled down the icy sidewalk, the snow blowing horizontally into our faces. This probably seemed like a silly, vain, and even dangerous thing to do. But to anyone who knows how important small, symbolic gestures are on the road to recovery, it was the most rational thing in the world. There was no way I was going to let her bail out on that hair appointment.

Another highlight from the past year: Mary Ann and I did something special last spring. For the first time in almost four years of marriage, most of it intertwined with our respective health struggles, we were finally able to take a real, old-fashioned vacation together. Yup, a week in Sedona, Arizona, with no agenda other than to relax, hike, explore the beautiful Southwest, poke around shops, be plain old tourists. Bought a beautiful hand-made pot from a Navajo woman by the side of the road. Even went horseback riding. It was a delight.

The hiking in Arizona is smooth and easy compared to rugged New England. Even so, Mary Ann was still walking gingerly. I had always dreamed of showing her the Grand Canyon, still the most spectacular place I've ever seen. But as we hiked down the Kaibab Trail, I could tell the pain and fear of falling was distracting her from fully enjoying the scenery. We didn't go too far.

Sure enough, not long after we got home, she had to have another knee surgery to help repair some of the lingering damage in there - her sixth surgery!

When I took her home from the hospital, she was all bandaged up and had to lay in bed with her leg elevated, and I kept changing her ice pack and bringing her tea, and she felt nauseous from the pain meds so I put a bowl beside her bed just in case, and it all seemed like déjà vu all over again. I was quietly heartbroken.

But guess what? She recovered incredibly fast. Before long she was walking with a surprising spring in her step, and was back to cracking her jokes - maybe the most encouraging sign of all. I guess maybe we were just getting good at all this.

179

Fast forward a few months later to another highlight, once again from the mountains in our back yard. This past October some friends invited us to join them on a hike up Mt. Washington, the tallest peak in the region. Way back in the summer of '09, after the surgery in which Dr. Trauma rebuilt Mary Ann's ankle, she asked if he thought she'd ever be able to climb Mt. Washington again. He did not give her an encouraging answer. I know that gnawed at her ever since...

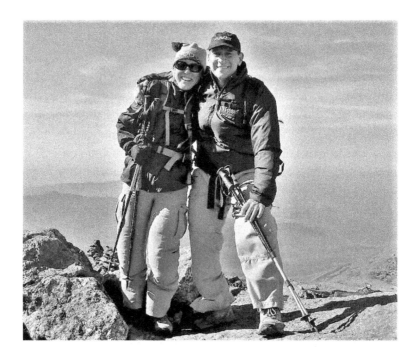

So here we were in October, both feeling pretty good, the weather forecast unusually mild, so we said why not? Let's see how far we get. We trudged up the Jewell Trail at a slow pace, more for my sake than Mary Ann's. (I've been having lung problems and I get out of breath easily.) After a couple hours, we emerged above treeline into the spectacular Alpine zone, then scrambled across the rocky terrain. Mary Ann would surge ahead, and then wait every so often for me to catch up. Before long we were standing at the summit, 6,288 feet above sea level, hanging on in the 60-MPH winds typical up there. It was our first time up there in four years. I can't even begin to describe the joy we felt on top of that rocky peak.

Then in typical Mary Ann fashion, she celebrated in another way: She had me take a publicity photo of her company's iPhone app functioning perfectly atop the Northeast's highest peak. I'm married to an absolutely relentless marketer!

So I've spoken about my mother and Mary Ann. You might be curious to know how *I've* been doing this past year, my third and now into my fourth year post-transplant. Relatively speaking, I guess I've come through the whole transplant and recovery process quite well. And there haven't been any signs that my leukemia or any related blood cancer is returning.

Even so, I still have some lingering little side effects from the treatment, and even more from an ongoing case of Graft-Versus-Host. These have led to a variety of issues with liver, tooth decay, achy muscles, cramping, and outbreaks of skin cancer (fortunately not the dangerous kind). None of these things have been major – they're more like minor irritants that I can certainly deal with. More troubling have been continuing difficulties with my lungs and dry eyes.

Sometimes the accumulation of all these things gets frustrating. So do all the doctors' appointments and trips to the pharmacy and baffling array of prescriptions drugs I have to take. Occasionally I get disappointed that I haven't been able to get anywhere near back to my former levels of strength and energy. It quietly kills me when I get exhausted carrying in a bag of groceries, or when I just run out of gas in the middle of the day. But like so many aspects of this whole journey, a lot depends on how you look at things. To paraphrase our friend Leonard Cohen, ring the bells that still can ring. And in the big scheme of things, I guess I'm ringing them relatively well.

One of the biggest highlights of the past year (actually of this whole journey) occurred in August while I was on a business trip to Los Angeles. I finally got to meet my donor Eric Rothman - the college student who donated some of his bone marrow stem cells to save my life. Looked him up and we met for a nice dinner overlooking the harbor in Marina Del Ray. He hasn't been able to land his dream sportscasting gig, but he's working for an agency that raises money for Israel. He seems to be settling nicely into life in LA, making friends, playing in basketball and softball leagues, and apparently he has a new girlfriend!

Here's a photo from our dinner. I was hoping I'd get some of Eric's thick crop of hair, but so far no such luck!

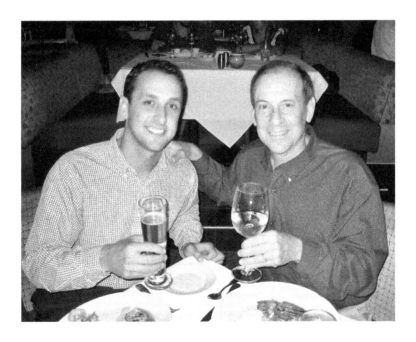

Anyway, it was a wonderful evening. How do you find the words to properly say thank you to a guy who did something like that? I hardly tried - he knew how grateful I felt. Better just to hang out together and talk about sports and life and the future.

———— ◦ ————

Not all of the last year has consisted of remarkable recoveries, triumphant summit hikes, and happy dinners. We've had our fair share of ups & downs with real-world stuff like work and health insurance and finances. I'd like to start by talking a bit about Mary Ann's work, because her story is a remarkable saga of tribulation and persistence.

Since returning to her career in broadcast equipment sales, she's been flourishing. Recently she was recognized with a promotion to Vice President, a rare title in her industry. When she told me the news, my first question was sort of crass - you can guess what I asked. That's right, how much of a raise did you get? Actually it wasn't much. It's a small company with relatively low pay to match. But then I realized how much this gesture meant to Mary Ann – in particular the sense of being valued and appreciated. And I know that in part it was a form of redemption after her career detour with our resort's real estate developers.

I've written about that whole episode in earlier entries, usually in restrained terms. But I think it's time to come out and be more blunt about what went on there. Why now, after so much time has passed and Mary Ann has moved so far beyond? Well maybe I just need to finally get all this off my chest as another step in moving on. But maybe more importantly, I think there are all sorts of lessons in there about how companies treat their employees, especially when they and their families are dealing with health challenges.

The story of Mary Ann's real estate bosses could make a great business school case study on how to demotivate your talent. First, they didn't accept input - in fact they gave her grief almost every time she spoke up with a helpful suggestion or creative idea. They allowed unscrupulous

183

colleagues to siphon off her rightful commissions – in one case, a co-worker literally pushed her aside while she was on crutches to get at a potential prospect who walked into the office. They made snide comments about her injuries (suffered, by the way, while working extra time to help them make a big sale), implying that she was somehow milking the system to get on the disability dole, and complaining that her workers comp claim would raise their insurance rates.

Maybe most troubling of all, they rarely lived up to the "family values" they purported to believe in. Yes, at first the top executives were supportive and compassionate, and several continued to be wonderful all the way through. But as with so many organizations, some middle managers didn't exactly walk the talk. For example, when I was first diagnosed with cancer, Mary Ann's boss encouraged her to quit. She wouldn't give her time off to drive me down to the hospital the day I was admitted. Then she continued to give her a hard time when she'd come down to Boston to visit me during the darkest days of my hospital stay.

The whole time during or since, we never received a single card, call, or gesture of goodwill from any member of her sales management team. Not one ounce of appreciation for our offer to buy one of their first house lots. And I've already mentioned the colleague who told Mary Ann that I "deserved" my cancer because I was a Jew who hadn't "accepted" Jesus Christ. Yikes! I think Jesus himself would be the last person on earth to make such a mean-spirited statement.

And even so, in the midst of a crumbling economy, much of the time caring for a gravely ill husband, often on crutches and hobbled by pain, Mary Ann still managed to generate more leads, customer relationships, and sales than the whole rest of the team put together, and all this while her "superiors" were arrogantly mismanaging and overspending their way into oblivion.

A telling postscript: Those same developers were recently foreclosed upon and abruptly closed up shop, leaving aborted development scars upon our landscape, absconding with our "refundable" club deposits, and having been heard from no more.

That whole chapter with Mary Ann's real estate job still stings a bit, especially when we consider how it played out against the backdrop of our medical struggles. But like so many other challenges we've encountered along this journey, we've tried to find the positives, take away some lessons, and even have a few laughs. For example, nowadays we chuckle at one of their remaining signs that refers to their old real estate sales office as the "Story Center" – all the ironic connotations of that silly name now ringing more true than ever. We still treasure some great friendships we made through Mary Ann's co-workers and sales contacts. Maybe most importantly, we've sure been reminded of the importance of treating employees, co-workers, and customers (indeed everyone) with respect and simple human decency. In any type of organization. No matter their job level. No matter their background.

Anyway, despite Mary Ann's recent career accomplishments, her present company is still so small that almost every aspect of the North American operations falls on her shoulders. It's been draining. They're also unable to pay her anywhere near what she's worth. Yes, the recognition is nice, but let's be realistic – the money is important too. Especially when I haven't been carrying my share of the financial load lately.

This gets to the heart of maybe the biggest strain of our past year. My corporate training work has continued to be sporadic, and I haven't been bringing in as much income as before I got sick (and before the economy crashed). At the same time, our health care bills have skyrocketed since my COBRA coverage expired this past summer. It's been an eye-opening experience trying to find coverage with my pre-existing condition of cancer. Some insurers tell me to get lost - I guess all the provisions of Obamacare still haven't kicked in fully yet. At least New

Hampshire now has a high-risk exchange where they can't overtly deny me coverage anymore – that's a step in the right direction. But the costs are astronomical. For the plans that we can afford, the deductibles are huge and the coverages limited.

It has been so frustrating trying to navigate the unimaginable complexities of the health insurance "system" while managing to keep on top of our bills. I've spent countless hours on the phone trying to untangle incomprehendable coverages, confusing bills, and payment snafus. It drains so much energy. And do you know how humiliating it is – especially for a 58-year-old man who's been financially comfortable most of his life – to bounce a check or receive a notice from a collection agency about an unpaid hospital bill that somehow slipped through the cracks?

While Obamacare certainly isn't perfect, I applaud the President for recognizing our country's health care mess and trying to do something about it. And frankly, it pisses me off to hear so many pundits and politicians spewing out empty rhetoric and misinformation just to score political or ideological points – that doesn't do anything to help me or others in our situation, or for that matter our nation as a whole. I certainly don't have the answer. But I do know that our struggles with insurance coverage and medical bills have diverted a huge portion of our money, energy, and focus lately. Multiply that by all the other Americans struggling in the same way, and in many cases far worse, and I think it all adds up to a huge drain on our nation.

———◦———

Bringing this all down to a more personal level, I've had a huge insight lately. I mentioned above that most of our financial burdens have been falling increasingly on Mary Ann's shoulders. My big insight has been realizing how much *I've* done to let that happen. I guess I've just let the work side of my life drift along, sitting back and waiting for the economy to "pick up again." Without realizing it, I've settled into career inertia, even a rut of sorts. Yes, it's been easy to rationalize this by pointing fingers at the curtailed spending by my corporate clients, the health insurance mess, my miscellaneous medical issues, my advancing age, etc. Maybe at the most subconscious level, my original cancer itself has something to do with it, like some deep, hidden anchor weighing me down.

Well it really jolted me recently to hear both Mary Ann and my mother - totally independently of each other – each use the "V" word. Yes, they both cautioned me about seeing myself as a victim. Hearing that word was a real wake-up call.

…Way back when I was a lazy, day-dreaming teenager, my father Bob used to give me lectures/pep talks to get me motivated. He would frequently quote a phrase from Sartre to the effect of "Man is free to act, but man must act to be free," or something like that. Of course, at the time I just rolled my eyes and drifted back into my apathetic teenage languor.

But wow, has that phrase rung true recently. I cannot think of any advice that's more important for cancer survivors. Beware inertia and stagnation and ultimately atrophy – it can creep in silently, unnoticed. It can affect you in all sorts of different ways. You may have survived the initial onslaught of the disease, but you still might face ongoing physical challenges, financial challenges, career challenges, mental challenges, emotional challenges, even relationship challenges. Dealing with any of these takes initiative and work– you can't just drift along.

I'd even say to be careful of the word "survivor" itself. While it certainly has a wonderfully positive meaning on the surface, at a subconscious level it may imply that you've made it through the big climax and now you can coast. It's sort of like a football team that builds a big lead in the third quarter and then lets down on offense. (Maybe I'm projecting my frustration with the way the Patriots played too many times this past season!) Yes, there's a time to accept your limitations gracefully. But there's also a time to keep striving, to keep playing offense. Going back to that phrase I've used from Leonard Cohen about "ringing the bells that still can ring," well they don't ring by themselves – you still have to pull the rope.

Well enough of my mixed metaphors. I recently made a decision that might seem illogical in light of what I just said about our financial challenges. For the last couple winters, I've been thinking about a few of my ski instructor buddies who went above and beyond the call of duty when I was really sick. I'll always remember their simple gestures: phone calls, cards, offers to do errands, jokes, pranks, and prayers. I'll never forget the time I was curled up on the bed feeling pretty low, and the phone rang and it was a strain just to reach over and pick it up, and it was from RJ and a group of instructors calling from the middle of the ski slope across the street, and when I hoisted myself up to look out the window, I could see them all waving their ski poles in the air. That was one of the most touching sights I've ever seen.

I've been wondering about a proper way to say thank you, and I think I've found it. Later this winter, I'm going to take a few of my instructor friends on a guys-getaway ski trip to Montana. Maybe it's not the most pragmatic thing to do. But as I've said before, not everything makes practical sense during these journeys. Sort of like my mother's hair appointment.

Mary Ann and I made another other similarly illogical decision recently. Mostly at her urging, we decided to take a trip to Israel. She's always dreamed of taking me there. In the midst of our respective health struggles the last few years, somehow we've managed to rack up a lot of airline and hotel points, especially her. After all we've gone through, both work and health-wise, we felt it was finally time to cash in those points and do something really special together. So we did, and here we are.

…And that finally brings me back to the moment, sitting alone in the now-quiet concierge lounge of the Tel Aviv Renaissance Hotel. I've been here for many hours, still pecking away at the computer. The last glow of sunset faded long ago, the Mediterranean is dark. The lounge staff has taken away the last of the evening sweets, and they've already set up for the morning's breakfast. I'm exhausted from our long day of being tourists today, but I just want to get all this typed in (at least in rough note form) - especially the part where I tell you about our amazing day today, and what motivated me to write all this. So here goes:

Mary Ann said that Israel would change me, and boy was she right. I won't bore you with a standard travelogue listing all the places we've visited. In short, Israel is a vibrant place rich in history and culture. We've been staying in Tel Aviv, a bustling, cosmopolitan city, surprisingly secular. Filled with all types of people, sports, teeming outdoor markets, and great food. Oh yes, cute women, too – I especially like the young ladies in military uniforms with automatic rifles dangling from their hip. Mary Ann always gives me a good-natured wise crack when she catches me checking them out!

Today we visited Jerusalem, an entirely different environment from Tel Aviv. More serious, intense. Surprisingly hilly. The old section of Jerusalem took us back in time. We walked through narrow cobblestone streets lined with merchants selling rugs and jewelry and spices. We wandered through Jewish, Arab, and Christian neighborhoods, each blending together with no apparent borders or signs. We saw Roman ruins, the spot where Jesus was crucified, the place where Mohammed rose to heaven, and all sorts of holy sites from Judaism – a mind boggling concentration of religion and history.

But two places today really stood out. Far beyond mere tourist destinations, they touched me deeply.

First was a visit to the Western Wall, formerly known as the Wailing Wall. I've always known it to be a spiritually and historically significant place for Jews, but not being much of a religious practitioner, I didn't know much more than that. Of course I wanted to visit it, just as I'd want to visit any historic site. So we walked with the throngs down the long series of steps into the plaza containing the Western Wall. I felt more like a tourist than a pilgrim. This was only heightened by all the pious looking guys we encountered along the walkway. They greeted me (while ignoring Mary Ann), put a hand on my forehead and offered some sort of blessing; with the other hand they held out their palm requesting an offering, into which I dutifully dropped the obligatory shekel (Israeli coin). Mary Ann and I both rolled our eyes and laughed as we continued down the steps, trying to weave through the gauntlet of outstretched palms in what we jokingly called the "Western Wall shakedown."

When we finally got down to the plaza, there was a wall separating the women from the men. (It's interesting how so many of the traditions of Orthodox Jews and Muslims are similar.) Mary Ann and I got whisked off in different directions. I followed the guy traffic through the plaza, and suddenly I was standing in front of this huge wall built of large rectangular stones. It seemed about the same size and scale as if I were standing in front of Fenway Park's Green Monster leftfield wall. I don't mean to be irreverent – that was honestly my first impression!

Suddenly I noticed how hushed and quiet it was, much like when you walk into a cathedral. Several guys were rocking back and forth praying, others touching the wall with their heads bowed, as if in a trance. There's a tradition there of writing little notes and prayers on a scrap of paper, and then placing it into the cracks between the stones. I wrote mine, and when I looked for a place to put it, I was amazed at how many other scraps were there – virtually every crack was jammed full. As I stuffed my note in, at first it felt like tossing a coin into a wishing well.

But then I touched the wall. As I held my palm against the stone, I felt a warmth. Not just the warmth of the sun on the stone, but a deeper warmth that spread up my arm and through my whole body. It transported me back to our first meeting with Dr. Soiffer - when he told us my best chance of survival was to get a bone marrow transplant from a matching donor, and because of my heritage, that donor had to be an Ashkenazi Jew. In the warmth of that stone, I felt the presence of Eric Rothman, an Ashkenazi Jew who donated his marrow to save my life. And I felt as if I was touching countless other Jews the world over. I felt a sudden connectedness with millions of people, throughout the centuries, just trying to help each other get by. It sent a warm shudder through my body, and I felt my world change a little…

The second place that made such an impression on me today was the Holocaust Museum. You can imagine what that was like, especially in a place like Jerusalem. All the expected displays and artifacts: Harsh public notices rounding up "Juden," touching diary entries and love letters, a chilling section of an actual boxcar that looked as if was designed to transport cattle, frayed blue-striped uniforms from concentration camps, and one jaw-dropping photograph of a man cradling his baby daughter to shield her from a German soldier about to fire a rifle at his head.

But the most powerful exhibit of all, the thing that really shook me to my core, was a video projected on a huge wall. It was a grainy black and white movie of families strolling, kids playing, couples walking hand in hand, seemingly in some picturesque eastern European town - very lifelike and peaceful and idyllic. Then we learned how it was made. It was composed of thousands of photos that were found in the wallets of people on their way to the death camps. Somehow the faces from these photos - people who ended up perishing in the Holocaust - were digitally combined with films of living people. For a second it created the illusion that they had made it, that somehow they'd been given a second chance. Then the reality struck. Very powerful – very moving. Made me think why they had to die… What if they had lived, what their future would have been like… And of course, why have so many others in my own situation had to die, why did I get the chance to survive, and how can I make the most of it… I stood there transfixed in front of that screen for a long time…

…So that's why I had to write this epilogue. I hope you can see why.

Yes, Mary Ann said that Israel would change me. And boy was she right. I don't know how, I don't know what's ahead, I don't know what new twists and turns this journey will take. But I know that I'll never be the same after today.

I know that I'll always feel a deeper connectedness, not just with those of my own heritage, but with people of all types everywhere who've been dealt a tough hand, and who can use a little help and compassion to make it through.

I know that I'll appreciate and savor all the more the gift of life I was so fortunate to receive. I'll be forever committed to making the most of it, living out the true spirit of the Hebrew toast that has so come to life on this trip: "l'chaim," meaning "to life." Life with a capital L.

I'll be forever thankful to all those who've helped us along our journey. And I know that somehow, at least in some small, indirect ways, the rest of my life will be devoted to returning the favor. Who knows, maybe this story will even help.

Part 8

TRANSITIONS

Time to do this

This time, RJ was right on *my* tail. But unlike four years ago, no snow was spraying from our skis, and no one was whooping like a teenage boy. At least not yet. We were high above the massive ski resort of Big Sky, Montana, cautiously inching our way along a narrow cat-track with a terrifyingly steep drop about six inches to the right of our skis. "Watch for the bumps up ahead," I cautioned back to RJ. "I see a place we can drop in after that." I stopped at a little ledge and carefully swiveled my skis out over the lip. Between my ski tips I spotted Walter and Billy, antlike, a couple thousand feet below. It was so steep that I couldn't see what lay directly beneath me. *"OK, time to do this."* I took a deep breath and dropped over the edge.

The first couple turns were almost like freefalling. But then my skis started gripping, I gained control, and I let loose, joyfully arcing back and forth across the face. It was like dancing with gravity. I gradually scrubbed some speed and eased my way to a stop part way down. My heart was pounding from a combination of altitude, effort, and exhilaration. What a rush! I kept my celebratory fist pump small and subtle – any sudden move could trigger a slip down the steep slope. Carefully

193

I kicked a little step into the snow so I could turn uphill and watch RJ come down.

RJ had been there when I first returned to the slopes, 118 days after my transplant, watching from above as I tentatively snowplowed my way down the bunny slope. In fact, he'd been there from the moment I first got sick. Whether gathering a gaggle of instructors to wave from the ski slopes across the street when I was quarantined at home, or just calling every now and then to check in, beneath his gruff exterior RJ always found a way to show he cared. He'd had his own challenges, too. Now in his early seventies, he'd recently had *both* knees replaced. And now here he was, far above, perched on top of a sheer drop - another world of challenge from our gentle home hill back in Bretton Woods.

I craned my neck back to watch. He dropped over the edge. Within a few turns he found his balance, then got a nice rhythm going in that familiar RJ style. He came to a stop next to me, both of us clinging to the steep slope while exclaiming words like "awesome" and "pissah!" (That's a quirky New England term meaning great.) Only then did he tell me he'd never skied anything like that before. We made our way down to Billy and Walter, who were waiting in the more civilized terrain below, and the four of us frolicked our way down to the bottom. I'll never forget that run.

It always sounds a bit trite to say "give something back," but that's exactly what this trip was about. On the surface, it was simply a fun getaway for a group of middle-aged guys. But it was also a way to thank three of my ski instructor friends for their support and goodwill during my leukemia journey. So I cashed in a pile of airline points, arranged a nice condo on the slopes, and flew the gang out to enjoy some big mountain skiing in Montana. While we were out there, we didn't talk all that much about the core reason for the trip. Hey, we're guys, so most of the conversation focused on snow conditions and ski terrain and beer and, of course, the "scenery." But deep down everybody knew what the trip was all about.

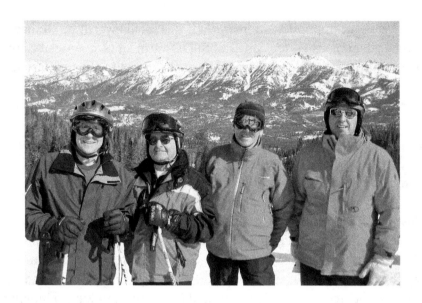

Earlier that winter I'd had an inkling that it might be my last season ski instructing. Our trip to Israel had stirred something deep within me - a subtle restlessness waiting to take form. Mary Ann and I were both feeling the first rumblings of evolving with our life, maybe even moving away from our beloved mountains. Deep down, I was also wondering if I'd hit a plateau in my recovery. I'd regained only part of my strength and stamina, my lungs were not so great, and maybe this was as good as it was going to get. And who knows how long even that would last. I'd been thinking about taking that ski trip for a long time. I'm glad I finally said "time to do this" and made it happen.

An interesting postscript: While we were out in Montana, they had a freak heat wave back in New Hampshire. When we returned home in early April, most of the snow had melted and our ski area had suddenly closed for the season – a few weeks earlier than expected. Had I not taken the initiative to book that trip, I wouldn't have had another chance to ski with the guys that season, and as it turned out, maybe ever.

Similar thing with my visit to my parents in Florida way back in April '09, a little over five months after my transplant. As soon as Dr. Soiffer gave me the OK to travel, I said "time do this" and booked the trip. I was still feeling pretty weak, and I had to wear a mask on the plane and out in public. No matter – it was totally worth it. We had a special, magical visit – tension-free, full of warm vibes, a sense of calmness now that I'd made it past the danger zone and life was settling back into place. My dad and I even went out on the tennis court and hit a few balls around. I'm not sure who had a harder time shuffling around the court, huffing and puffing, chasing after each other's errant shots. It was delightful. I'm so glad I took that trip and my parents got to see me on the road to recovery, especially my father. Four days after I returned home, he died suddenly.

Yes, the "time-to-do-this" lesson really resonates when you have a close brush with mortality - others' as well as your own. Cancer has a way of getting you thinking about stuff like that. You get more contemplative, reflective. You look at the little things, and you start connecting the dots. You look at the way you just drop over the edge of a ski run into the steep unknown below, and it gets you thinking. Thinking about decisions you made, and didn't make. Times you surged ahead, and times you played it safe. You wonder about that yin and yang of your life, and how it's all played out so far. You've made so many great moves, accomplished so many things, built such a rich, wonderful life... yet there's always been this nagging little voice of restraint, like an invisible hand tugging at your shirt tails, holding you back. Especially with your career. You've been adept at drifting along, making the best out of what comes your way, building the semblance of a successful work life. But you're still drifting. You get to thinking about that trip to Jerusalem and that video collage of Holocaust victims with their lives cut short, and you wonder what that feeling deep inside was all about, how to channel that restlessness into something meaningful. There's a purpose out there somewhere. In there somewhere. You long to create something. Achieve something. Amount to something. Make yourself proud. Make your wife proud. Help others. Move others. Reinvent yourself. Find yourself. Be yourself...

You decide to write a book. To start another chapter of your life and see where it takes you. To plunge off another ledge into the unknown. Time to do this.

At the peak

Physically, that fourth year post-transplant did indeed turn out to be the high point in my recovery. I was able to handle the rugged ski terrain of Big Sky without too many problems – just a stop for breath every so often and a couple rest days mixed in. Back in New Hampshire that summer, the same thing on the tennis court. It had taken a few years, but I was back to playing those vigorous points, sprinting side to side, leaping and lunging. It was a joy. Even so, after a hard point I'd find myself doubled over, gasping for breath. My tennis friends were always patient, calmly saying "take your time" before starting the next point. Hell, they probably appreciated the rest themselves!

Another thing during this period, far more important than my tennis game: I learned to be comfortable asking for a break – that was a big step forward.

I particularly enjoyed my frequent singles matches with our neighbor Daniel. On the court, our play was ferocious, filled with smashes and crashes, grunts and groans. Daniel was a bull – he'd charge after every shot, often crashing into the fence alongside the court. To tell the truth, I got a kick out of slicing those wide shots that ended up denting the fence – hey, I had to use every weapon I could! Only thing is, he'd bounce right off and get to my next shot, stretching, leaping, often smashing it back. We played hard. Daniel never let up. I loved it. I felt alive.

Like my other friends, he was always great about letting me take rest breaks. And believe me, after some of our crazy points, my lungs really needed it! When we switched sides after every other game, we'd sit on the bench and chat while my pulse rate calmed down. We had lots to talk about: Our latest hiking exploits; our constant struggles to maintain the great mountain views in our condo village; his challenges raising two teenage boys. Daniel was a professor of atmospheric science at Harvard. It was fascinating to hear about his research projects with NASA and NOAA, and to learn about the actual science behind climate change – what a refreshing change from all the political nonsense swirling around. He'd ask about my work in corporate education, which triggered heated discussions (and even debates) about best practices for teaching. Like most of our part-time neighbors, Daniel came up from his other life in the "real world" and infused our mountain retreat with worldliness and vitality. I always appreciated the stimulating conversation as much as the rigorous exercise.

On the medical front in year four, my blood counts had stabilized. My platelets were in the normal range, which meant my blood was able to clot effectively. My red cell counts had reached a plateau slightly below normal. This may be partially why I felt a little sluggish and out of breath, though Dr. Soiffer said not to worry about it. He felt my lungs were more of a concern. My white blood counts were in the normal range, which meant my immune system was at full strength.

One caveat, however, was that a too-strong immune system could exacerbate my graft-vs-host disease. In effect, my new immune system would keep attacking the old cells in my body. So I had to take an immune suppressant drug to keep those attacks in check. Dr. Soiffer regularly monitored my GVHD symptoms and tampered with my medications accordingly. It was a constant dance to maintain the right balance. This had become the central focus of my post-transplant care, and most likely will continue to be for the rest of my life. No tidy endings there.

On the other hand, there were no signs of any blasts or cancerous blood cells returning. At least in that regard, you could say I was cancer free.

While I've never been great at math, I've always loved numbers. From mountain elevations and weather data to economics and sports statistics, I've always found clarity and meaning in numbers. That's certainly true with medical metrics too, such as blood counts and pulse rates and pulmonary function readings and even mortality statistics. At my regular check-ups with Dr. Soiffer, we always huddle around the monitor as he reviews and interprets my latest blood lab results. Numbers have helped keep my cancer journey grounded in objectivity.

You've probably noticed that I've also used another, less quantitative type of metric to track my health: outdoor sports, especially hiking. And as for our hiking in that peak year of 2012, Mary Ann and I kept up the momentum from our triumphant climb of Mt. Washington the preceding fall. While nowhere near the speed and ambitious terrain of years before, I was able to sustain a moderate pace, huffing and puffing, taking a rest stop now and then. Mary Ann's ankle and knee had improved, and she'd regained her form on the trails. That was great to see. Always strong and relentless, she'd surge way ahead of me on the uphills. Downhill was a different story. Because it didn't tax my lungs, I'd practically skip my way down, while she went slowly and carefully, protecting her ankle on the rocky terrain.

Now that was a switch - Mary Ann the more deliberate one of us! But I guess there's a metaphor there of our life together: Taking turns sharing the lead, each with different roles, different strengths, different styles, striving for synergy, the push and pull of our differences not always easy, but hopefully all coming out, on balance, for the better. (Whew, what was that I said earlier about being contemplative?)

On the work front in Year Four, I was feeling better, too. Travel was no problem. My issues with cramps and dry eyes were irritants, not impediments. I was back to my old self in the workshops, not only drawing energy from the learners, but creating some of it myself. Even so, as with everything else, I'd need a rest every so often. Often that would mean quiet room service dinners in my hotel room instead of evening jaunts out on the town. Or a few days or sometimes even weeks at home between work trips.

The latter came automatically, as my work volume was still struggling to climb back from the recession. I rode along with it, always able to fill the slow periods with ski instructing and community activities. At the time, I appreciated how busy and varied my life was. In hindsight, however, I wonder if there was a little post-cancer rationalization mixed in there; maybe I was doing some of that dreaded drifting I mentioned earlier.

Mary Ann and I had also reached a peak of sorts in our social and community lives. Again through the perspective of hindsight, I realize we'd made an interesting transition. In the first difficult years of our intertwined health struggles, the Bretton Woods community had been a great source of support to us. But ever since then, you could say we'd been trying to return the favor. For example, I revamped and maintained our homeowner website, planned various community service events, and helped push for resort-wide shuttle service. Mary Ann co-led several homeowner golf tournaments that raised money for wounded veterans. We got involved organizing all sorts of benefits and parties, constantly striving to enrich our community from within. It was very satisfying, a touch therapeutic, and a hell of a lot of fun.

One of my fondest memories was a big community party we organized that also served as a food drive for needy people in the area. (And believe me, when you got away from our little upscale resort enclave, there sure were many needy folks up there in the North Woods.) Among a zillion other duties, Mary Ann ended up playing bartender that night. This mainly consisted of filling people's wine glasses and handing bottles of beer over the bar counter. I hope she doesn't kill me for saying this, but she looked spectacular – in particular, she was wearing a fetching dress that was a bit low-cut in the front. Well let me just say that the beer consumption that night was huge, especially among the guys! Her tip jar filled to the brim, too!

And as for Mary Ann, well she'd sure come a long way from that scrawny, bespectacled bookworm who played cello in the school orchestra and immersed herself in books so she wouldn't have to talk to anyone. I'll always remember the laughs and friendship and good cheer of that night as the pinnacle of our wonderful community life in Bretton Woods. And by the way, of course Mary Ann donated all her tips to the food drive.

Farewell to the mountains

You know how when you open an ap on your smartphone or a new website on your PC, the old one disappears underneath? It's still running, but now hidden below the surface. Well, by 2012 that's sort of what had happened with our respective health struggles. Whereas they'd been at the forefront of our lives for several years, they'd now receded into the background, still there, but below the surface. In short, we had reclaimed control of our lives.

Sometimes big decisions don't come in a single flash, but rather in dribs and drabs, like a leaking faucet when the drips start sounding louder and louder. We started hearing drips: The constant trudges through windblown snowdrifts to scrape windshields and free ice-encrusted wiper blades. Watching the Academy Awards and realizing we hadn't seen any of the Best Picture nominees. The half-hour drives to buy groceries or pick up my prescriptions. The three-hour treks down to Boston for my numerous medical appointments. All those late-night drives back home from the Manchester airport, droopy eyelids fighting to scan for dark shapes in the road; Mary Ann stumbling home one night in particular at 3:30 am, traumatized and shaking after a dark, foggy, sleet-slicked drive through the empty mountains. Petty squabbles over miniscule issues like flower beds and tree trimming erupting into major conflicts, way out of proportion, tarnishing our community's little peace of paradise. (Yes, I meant to spell it that way.) The menu at good old Fabyan's starting to get a bit stale, and our regular seats at the bar - while always a wonderful source of familiarity and comfort - also becoming a vantage point to observe the same après-ski crowd and the same bar chatter, the same rhythms and routines of the resort lifestyle.

Yes, Bretton Woods was a great getaway destination - an amazing place to play, connect, enrich, and recharge. And we'd had a wonderful run there building our life together while maintaining full-time careers. That was rare among the handful of full-timers up there – most were retirees. But we were still working, growing, striving, looking ahead. And speaking of looking ahead, who knew what was in store for our health, especially mine. Well, those bar stools at Fabyan's gave us a look in the mirror and a glimpse into our future. We realized it was time for a change. And now, when we were at the top of our game, was the time to make it happen.

We explored the Maine coast, and fell in love with the hip bustle of Portland. The restaurants, theaters, stores, culture, and airport so close. Just outside of town, we discovered beautiful beaches, bucolic farmland, and quaint white-steeple villages – like New England post cards at every turn. Our realtor took us through one such village, Yarmouth, to view a unique-looking house we'd seen on line. The second we drove up the driveway, we were captivated by the place's character and potential. It was a bit run-down and overgrown, but we saw a diamond in the rough. As I scanned the heavily wooded yard, I dreamed of cutting our own firewood and sculpting the land into a work of natural beauty. When Mary Ann walked inside, her first reaction was a big, beaming smile and a single word in German: "gemütlichkeit!" It's hard to find an English synonym, but it means something like warm, cozy ambiance. We were smitten. Change beckoned. Time to do this. We made the deal.

Our Bretton Woods neighbors threw a goodbye party for us, and 35 people showed up. The running joke, with which we played right along, was that it was more of a good riddance party!

It wasn't easy saying goodbye to the great community, wonderful friends, outdoor fun, inspiring scenery, and that incredible night sky. Like the mountains all around, my 12 years in Bretton Woods had been full of peaks and valleys, which only enriched my experience living there: From the early years as a fun weekend getaway, to a place of lonely exile; the place where I pieced my life back together; the place I married the love of my life; the place we started building a promising future together; the place where it all came crashing down; and the place that helped nurture us back. I sometimes wonder if it all would have played out the same anywhere else - I even wonder if Bretton Woods in some small ways helped save my life. In any case, it certainly was the place where I was reborn... twice! I'll always treasure that.

Welcome to Maine

So there we were, the first time we discovered our little local beach, a short bike ride from our new home. It wasn't much of a beach, just a strip of sand that expanded and contracted with the tides. I was barefoot, as I always like to feel the sand and slosh through the salt water. Mary Ann wore her sandals. We strolled along the shoal that emerged from the receding tide, reaching down every now and then to pick up a shell or piece of sea glass. The orange sunset reflected across the bay. Seagulls cackled overhead. There was a soft warm breeze. I can't even remember who said it aloud first, but as we so often do, virtually in unison our minds latched onto the same thought: "Geez, why were we so snarky when we made fun of those on-line dating phrases? These 'walks-on-the-beach' are pretty nice after all!" Of course, that launched us into a playful back-and-forth banter as we strung together one corny dating cliché after another. So typical. So wonderful. So much a part of what I love about her...

———◦———

I've long thought about a concept that I call the theory of pendulum swings. By this I mean that things trend toward one extreme, then that causes a reaction to swing the pendulum back in the opposite direction, and so forth. It certainly applies in politics, with power swinging back and forth between the parties. Also at deeper levels, such as the constant tug of war between free enterprise and government intervention, and so on.

Well before I get too carried away (and in over my head) here, let me bring it down to a more personal level. Our move to Maine was like a pendulum swing to another type of world. We savored the differences, appreciated the little things that one might otherwise take for granted. For example, there was a supermarket less than a mile away - during our first couple weeks, Mary Ann must have gone over at least three times a day! Nearby was a dry cleaner and a bank and a Chinese restaurant and, maybe most convenient of all, a Rite Aid pharmacy. A little ways beyond that, my own personal mecca: a Home Depot. We could get to (and home from) the airport in minutes rather than hours. To us, these seemed like godsends.

After so many years in a remote mountain resort, we now lived in a real neighborhood. Kids played in the streets and gathered for the school bus and, as it would soon turn out, rang our doorbell on Halloween. We loved it.

Inside and out, the house needed lots of updating. There was so much character there, just waiting to be unleashed. We plunged right in, scraping off the hideous flower-print wallpaper, and painting over the dreary colors from yesteryear. It wasn't easy. For every layer of wallpaper we removed, it seemed another sprung to life underneath. Every wall we painted took coat after coat to hide the old dark colors. Far more things needed repairing or replacing than we noticed when we first saw the place. It didn't take long to realize that we were in for a long, multifaceted rehab adventure. But we were energized by all the projects, and thrilled with each little step forward.

Our overgrown yard was full of potential, and now I had the freedom to cut a tree or two with nobody freaking out that I was "mutilating Mother Nature." (Yes, someone in Bretton Woods actually said that.) I started attacking the messy yard. One of the first tasks was to remove a huge clothesline in full view of the street out front. Typical of the previous owner, who over-built everything, the clothesline was massive. It consisted of two t-shaped crosses made from heavy lumber posts, each embedded in concrete deep underground. After several hours of toil, I finally managed to dig out one of the end pieces and started hauling it out back to cut it up. Apparently Mary Ann had quite a chuckle when she looked out her office window and saw this Jewish guy slowly trudging through the yard, bent over under the weight of a massive wooden cross on his back!

The overall vibe in Maine was more agrarian than the NH mountains, with local cheese and produce and microbrews available everywhere. Great seafood too, often right off the boat. Nearby was the flagship store of the iconic LL Bean; the whole area seemed like their catalog come to life. Everyone was always out walking or jogging, usually with a dog in tow (or vice versa). We bought nice road bikes, and cycling replaced hiking as our new sport of choice.

Fifteen minutes away, downtown Portland teemed with art galleries and theaters and cool restaurants and coffee shops. When we went into town, Mary Ann starting playfully fancying herself as an "urban hipster" - I guess another type of pendulum swing away from her totally uncool school days.

One more thing about our move to Maine – a huge one: It brought us an hour closer to Boston, and all my medical facilities and doctors down there. Also closer to my brothers and their families, and especially to my mother. That was reassuring in many ways.

My mother helped us decorate and furnish the new place. She has great taste, and she added a unique sense of style to our house. But this was about so much more than decor. It warmed my heart to see Nancy and Mary Ann bonding over paint colors and rugs and jaunts to the local antique stores. And when the two of them would get a bit carried away with form, I'd speak up as the voice of function. We each had our roles. We made a good team. It was exciting to see our house slowly start to transform, room by room, each refreshed and renewed. Maybe a bit like our life?

Our renovation project was satisfying in another way, too. It seemed to reinvigorate Nancy by giving her a sense of purpose. That's very important to a widow in her mid-80's. Come to think of it, it's important to anyone. Purpose is healthy.

Part 9

YEAR FIVE DOWNTURN

A sudden slide down

I've already mentioned several times how cancer journeys are rarely linear. You can always expect twists and turns, ups and downs, steps forward and back, etc. Well, my fifth and sixth years post-transplant, 2013-14, sure proved that to be the case. Along with the excitement of our new home and life in Maine, my health took a turn for the worse. A lot worse.

First of all, let me answer the question that everyone always thinks but is uncomfortable asking: No, there were still no signs of my cancer returning. My basic blood readings remained OK - stable and acceptable, if not perfect. That's the key yardstick of my cancer, and in that way I was still doing fine.

But leukemia isn't always as simple as that. Post-transplant recovery is often accompanied by all sorts of after effects and side effects. And not long after our move to Maine, all of mine seemed to flare up at the same time. Apparently, the main cause was a spike in my Graft vs. Host disease. Dr. Soiffer explained that's often the case with chronic GVHD patients like me. I also speculated whether some of the long-term effects (or "collateral damage," to use the military term) from my radiation treatments years earlier may have been kicking in. I wondered if leaving our vigorous mountain lifestyle may have played a part. Or could it even have had something to do with our new house itself? Who knows? Whatever the cause, I started feeling crappy in more ways than I can count. It was like getting pummeled from so many different directions that you finally start to wilt.

Part of me is hesitant to share the details. It'll sound like a long list of gripes, and the last thing I want to do is be a complainer or whiner or anything like that. After all, I'd beaten the odds of even being alive at this point, and beyond that, I was relatively active and (mostly) functional. Can't take that for granted. Even so, this setback was an important and difficult phase of our journey, with multiple offshoots, so I want to try to paint a picture of what it was like.

Somewhere during this period, I started noticing that I had to tighten my belt an extra notch to hold my pants up. Mary Ann teasingly started calling me "Mr. No-Ass." One day I was in a hotel room about to take a shower. The room had a closet with folding doors that were mirrors. The doors were partially open, creating reflections from unusual angles. As I walked past the closet, I was startled to see a man standing there! He looked scrawny, almost skeletal, with a sunken chest and shoulder bones poking through his skin. It was me! Seeing myself from that unfiltered perspective was a jolt.

When I got home and stepped on a scale (something I rarely did), I was shocked to see that my weight had dropped into the 140's! That was less than my weight ever dipped during the lowest points of my transplant and its aftermath. In fact, I hadn't weighed that little since college, over forty years earlier; I recalled that when I was on the soccer team, I asked them to fudge my weight on the program up to 150 pounds so I wouldn't seem like such a lightweight. (Yeah, right. Like those other players must have sure been intimidated when they saw that Gordon dude weighed all of 150!) Anyway, here I was in middle age - the time when most men are struggling with rotund bellies that roll over their belt buckles – and I looked almost emaciated.

Even more alarming, most of my weight loss seemed to be from losing muscle mass, and thereby strength. I started to have difficulty with outdoor tasks such as chain sawing and raking. I had to fill the wheel barrow only halfway in order to be able to push it. Indoors, simple chores like painting overhead and even turning a screwdriver became a strain. Once I was boarding a flight and struggled to lift my roller case into the overhead compartment – a woman standing in the aisle had to reach over and give me a hand. That was humbling. My regular push-up routine declined to the point where I could barely do one or two. It was scary to wonder if something inside me was eating away at my muscles.

My muscles weren't just getting weak, but also achy and stiff, often numb, almost paralyzed. I started getting severe cramps all over. These became much more than annoyances - they prevented me from doing everyday tasks. Bending down to tie my shoes would trigger abdominal cramps, leaving me doubled over in pain for several minutes. My hands would often seize up, which twisted my fingers into disfigured knots and prevented me from holding a pen or typing or even reading a book. Cramps in my lower legs would keep me tossing and turning at night. Most excruciating of all were the hamstring cramps in the back of my thighs. They'd hit without warning, often dropping me to the floor writhing and groaning, sometimes even screaming. I'm really not being dramatic here – that's exactly how it went. The cramps were brutal, and the hardest part was not knowing when or where they would strike.

My dry eye problems got worse, too. Like my cramps, the flare-ups were not only irritating and painful – they affected my ability to function normally. In my training workshops, I'd strain to read the learners' name cards across the room or even my own notes in front of me. I felt self-conscious about how sunken and red my eyes looked, which affected my demeanor and confidence. That's what I meant by offshoots.

At the store, I couldn't read product labels or prices. Outdoors, sometimes the slightest breeze would irritate my eyes to the point where I had to close them - among many other activities, that made bicycling difficult. Occasionally I'd have a hard time driving. Maybe most frustrating of all was when my eye flare-ups would prevent me from reading – it's amazing how much that makes you feel cut off from the world. Another offshoot. There's got to be some irony in there somewhere to think that all this was related to my body's inability to manufacture tears.

One time my eyes were so irritated that I could only open my eyelids a crack, and what little I could see was a total blur. I found my way to the medicine cabinet and felt for a little bottle of eye drops. I pried open an eye and squirted in a drop. My eye exploded in searing pain. I flung the bottle away and covered my eyes with my hands. The stinging and burning were incredible - like my eye was on fire. There was nothing I could do – open them, close them, wet face cloth - nothing helped. I managed to put my head under the tap and run cold water over my eyes. It took about five minutes for the pain to subside to the point where I could open my eyes a crack and see (blurrily). Only then did I realize that I had mistakenly grabbed a bottle of ear wax remover and squirted it into my eye! Is it sick of me to look back on that now and think it was sort of funny? Well I do. But it sure wasn't funny at the time.

GVHD causes dryness not only in the eyes, but also in the skin. My skin constantly felt dry and raw, and sometimes it broke out in itchy rashes. My mouth dried out, too. Nights were the worst. I'd wake up several times each night with my mouth so parched that it felt like cotton. Often this was accompanied by a metallic, chemical taste. And this led to yet one more side effect: Without the proper amount of saliva in my mouth, which serves as an antibacterial agent, tooth decay set in, and my dental problems (and bills) mounted. More offshoots.

With all my countless blood tests ever since my transplant, the one area that's consistently been most out of whack has been my liver function readings. In part, this may be a byproduct of my initial radiation treatments, though that's just my own speculation. I do know that post-transplant GVH disease often targets the liver, and apparently it messed up mine. From what I've learned, the liver controls a wide variety of functions such as removing toxins, secreting hormones and enzymes, aiding digestion, and maintaining overall body chemistry. I wonder if that's why so many things have felt a little "off" over the years.

Possibly related to my liver issues, my stomach problems flared up during this period. Aches, burning, churning, occasional nausea. Evenings were particularly tough, curled up on the couch watching TV with Mary Ann. What should have been a relaxing time was often interrupted by the sounds of my gurgling and belching and groaning with discomfort. Mary Ann was always understanding and a good sport about it, but I know it grated on her.

Various GI and UT issues arose, too. I'd rather not go into the details, and you probably don't want to hear them anyway. Let's just leave it that it wasn't pleasant.

You already know that I'd had some mild lung problems ever since my initial diagnosis. But during this tough stretch in years five and six, my breathing got a lot worse. It's hard to describe exactly - it was much more than just huffing and puffing. A short burst of exertion would send a strange burning sensation through me, deadening my muscles and leaving me gasping for breath, often weak and dizzy to the brink of fainting. That was hard enough when I was trying to shovel a snowy path or rake a flower bed – but much worse when cycling up a long hill with cars whizzing past and my bike starting to wobble. Our joyous climb of Mt. Washington now seemed like a lifetime ago, totally unthinkable at this point – I had a hard enough time making it up the 13 steps to our second-floor bedroom. Sometimes just a simple task like bending over to pick up a laundry basket would leave me panting and spent.

I did the best I could with my various activities, adjusting the pace and duration according to how I felt, and trying to accept my limitations gracefully. That helps you cope. But it's hard to do when you feel one of your greatest sources of joy slipping away.

One early winter day, when Mary Ann was away on a business trip, I decided to head over to a little local ski hill and try some skiing. I hadn't skied in a couple winters and was curious to see how I'd do. It wasn't a good sign when I struggled to lug my skis from the parking lot, and then could barely lean over to put on my ski boots. Once I finally made it onto the slopes, it wasn't pretty - and I'm not just talking about my skiing form. Everything hit me at once: stiff joints, weak muscles, lack of breath, cramps, irritated eyes, and more. I flailed my way down the slope like an out-of-control beginner, barely able to see, struggling to keep my balance, skidding awkwardly to a stop every couple hundred feet to catch my breath. I'd stand at the side of the slope hunched over my poles, gasping, dizzy, my legs trembling. After a few minutes, I'd try another stretch. Same result. I gave up after a couple runs. When I finally sat down in the base lodge, it was a ten-minute struggle just to lean over and pull off my ski boots without cramping or fainting.

For the rest of that winter, Mary Ann and I didn't ski together once.

Everything accumulated during this period. Overall, I felt increasingly sluggish and exhausted. It took a big effort to break the inertia and get moving. Then, with the slightest exertion, the fatigue would envelop me and drag me back down. I started taking lots of naps. That was a disheartening and even frightening feeling of déjà vu.

As if all these side effects weren't enough, I also had numerous outbreaks of skin cancer. Early on, Dr. Soiffer had suggested I get regular check-ups from a dermatologist, and that proved to be good advice. By being proactive, we caught most of the outbreaks early, many in a pre-cancerous stage; the dermatologist would usually just freeze them away or lop them off in her office. No big deal.

Several times the skin cancers progressed to the point where I needed a procedure called Mohs surgery. This is where they remove thin layers one at a time, and biopsy them right in the office – they keep going until all the cancer is gone. Again, no big deal, and in a wacky sort of way, I even found these procedures enjoyable. While they biopsy each layer, you get to hang out in a comfortable waiting room (properly bandaged and anesthetized, of course), reading, writing, and enjoying the free coffee and snacks. I guess it doesn't take much to amuse me.

Anyway, the good news with my skin cancers is that they were all the basal or squamous varieties – not that dangerous as long as we caught them early. The only byproduct so far has been little scars and pockmarks all over, which don't bother me in the least. In fact, I get a kick out of them – along with my many other scars from orthopedic surgeries, they're all sort of badges of honor. Lurking underneath, however, there's always the risk for more dangerous types of skin cancer to break out – then the story might be different. There's not much I can do about that except keeping up with my proactive dermatology checks, and slathering on sunscreen when I go outside. I won't stay indoors.

One of my skin cancer outbreaks led to an interesting side story. What had first appeared as an innocuous little spot on the top of my ear turned out to be the tip of a deep basal growth below - like an iceberg. The Mohs surgery doctor had to remove several layers to get it all out. Then he attempted to repair the site by grafting some skin from the back of my ear. Unfortunately, the graft didn't take. Over the next couple weeks, it turned into a black, decaying mess. I kept it hidden under a bandage when I was out in public. I called the doctor about it. He said he had a 98% success rate with his skin grafts, but unfortunately I must have been in the 2% group. (By the way, this was a great example of what I said earlier about finding numbers so helpful.) So he brought me back to remove the failed graft and discuss options for Plan B.

This doc was a great guy – warm, personable, with a humorous wit and a classic Boston accent. He was originally from Brockton, a small city south of Boston. We chatted about all the usual things you talk about if you've grown up in that area: long-forgotten Red Sox and Bruins players from years ago, memories of teenage runs to Friendly's and Dunkin Donuts, our favorite Aerosmith songs, and of course Brockton's special claim to sporting fame as the home of boxing greats Rocky Marciano and Marvin Hagler.

So there we were, chatting away as he scraped away the failed graft and dead skin from my numbed-up ear. Suddenly he asked "Hey Peter, got a strong stomach? Wanna take a look?" I always liked to be involved in my treatments, so I said sure. He handed me a mirror, and I held it up to the side of my head. *Holy shit!* I was shocked to see a bloody mess, with a huge semi-circular chunk of my ear missing. "Wow, it looks like Evander Holyfield's ear after the Tyson fight," I kidded. We both started exchanging jokes about Mike Tyson and that crazy boxing match. Humor can be its own type of anesthetic.

But underneath the banter, I was also doing a little mental

multi-tasking about the jolt I felt when I saw my ear. No, it wasn't the blood and gore itself – that didn't bother me. But rather what it represented: A visual manifestation of my cancer, like an exclamation point in bold font - a vivid reminder that years after my transplant, the effects continue, and a piece of me is missing. That got me thinking about what else I'd lost, would I ever get it back, and would I be disfigured forever - not physically, but in other, more meaningful ways... As I said before, you get contemplative about things, and your mind can take you many places in ten seconds while you're sitting in an exam chair jabbering about boxing.

Anyway, the Mohs doc said he wasn't confident he could repair it at this point, so he'd have to send me to another specialist. I found his directness and honesty refreshing. He referred me to a reconstructive surgeon, who ended up doing a great job putting my ear back together. Well, at least most of it – I didn't give her a lot to work with. For what it's worth, she shared the same engaging manner as the first doc – competent and confident enough to let a little personality and humor shine through. She did the best she could, though there's still a piece missing from the upper lobe. Just another badge of honor, as far as I'm concerned. I hardly even notice it anymore, but when I do, it gives me warm memories of my two ear surgeons.

And that's typical of this whole period. Intermixed with my physical problems, and sometimes even because of them, there were silver linings everywhere. For example, we thought we'd left the heavy mountain snows behind when we moved down to the coast, but no such luck - the winters in those years were brutal. But when our neighbor across the street saw me struggling to shovel the path or rake the roof or chop through the thick ice on the driveway, he'd come right over to lend a hand. That great bit of neighborly goodwill might not have happened otherwise.

In summer, all the tree cutting and brush piles were starting to get ahead of me - I just didn't have the strength or stamina to keep up. So our nephew Ben came up for a few days to trim tree limbs and haul brush and help with the firewood. There's an old saying that firewood warms you four times: cutting, splitting, stacking, and burning. Well I can add a fifth item to that list: getting to spend precious time with your nephew.

I experienced other silver linings from my bicycle seat. Our area was a road biking paradise, with classic Maine rocky coastline, pastoral farmland, and quaint white-steeple villages – often all on the same ride. Along the way, we'd discover great little roadside places to stop for a lobster roll or homemade ice cream. It was like a Yankee Magazine come to life. Yes, the pedaling was becoming a strain for me, and my pace slowed way down – but that allowed me to savor the local scenery and character all the more.

As my breathing and strength declined, my struggles on the bike got worse. The uphills were especially tough. I can't begin to describe how discouraging it was sometimes to have to get off my bike part way up a climb, doubled over panting and dizzy. Occasionally I'd even have to walk the rest of the way up the hill. That was painful, not least because I knew I was making Mary Ann wait for me somewhere up ahead.

But then again, to see her zipping ahead on her snazzy new carbon bike, her powerful legs pumping away like pistons - that gave me a little flutter of joy. I thought back to our first date, when I was the one sprinting ahead and she teasingly called me Lance... I thought back to her lying in a hospital bed with her leg all bandaged up from one of her many surgeries, hoping and praying that she'd be able to walk normally again... and now look at her go! I always got such a kick watching her surge ahead out of sight.

Yes, there were silver linings everywhere. We continued to discover great surprises about our new world on the Maine coast. We slowly made progress on the house and yard, one little rewarding step at a time. We savored relaxing with a glass of wine in front of our cozy fireplace. Or hanging out on our screened porch, sipping coffee and reading the paper, while the cats raced back and forth following the chipmunks and birds outside. We never stopped appreciating the wonderful moments.

But I'd be putting a falsely rosy spin on those years if I didn't say this was a difficult phase. Sure, it's always good to appreciate the silver linings; you certainly don't want to let the disappointments and frustrations blind you to the positives. On the other hand, it works in both directions. Silver linings don't cancel out the bad stuff, or sanitize the struggle. It's not a zero-sum game. Rather, it's a complex, constant juggling act, where you toggle back and forth between the good and bad in your mind, hoping to find a realistic, healthy balance. It takes mental effort, especially to keep toggling back to the positives when you feel the negatives weighing you down.

And that's exactly what was happening. My symptoms not only got more severe, but they'd come at me in multiple combinations, like a perfect storm. Sometimes they'd slow me way down, other times they'd stop me in my tracks. I felt like that mythological guy Sisyphus who keeps pushing the boulder up the hill, only to have it roll back down. Maybe worst of all was the unpredictability of when it would start to roll again. As I've said before, uncertainty is a huge burden in and of itself.

And as if my physical struggles weren't hard enough, the offshoots also reached out to other parts of our life, like tentacles, entangling us in other ways.

Offshoots and tentacles

Way back when, while we were waiting anxiously to find a donor for my transplant, I told you how I occupied myself by keeping meticulous records. Well I've continued that practice ever since. It's proven to be very helpful, especially for tracking medical expense deductions on our tax returns. Looking back on the data has also yielded some interesting insights into our healthcare journey. For example, during my post-transplant downturn in years five and six, Mary Ann and I made a total of 88 separate visits to various doctors and medical providers' offices. All but a handful of these were mine: skin doctor, lung doctor, cancer doctor, colon doctor, family doctor, urology doctor, eye doctors, skin surgeons, dentists, blood labs, radiology clinics, and I can't even remember what else. 88 trips! Add to that, another 54 trips to pharmacies to pick up prescriptions and medical supplies. Total miles driven for these 142 trips: 6,049. That's a lot of running around. A lot of offshoots.

The total time and effort was one thing, but there was another, less tangible effect - I guess you could call it the "opportunity cost" (a term I vaguely remember from business school). By this, I mean that all the running around diverts you from so many other things you could be doing; it breaks your momentum, and almost takes on a life of its own. In my case, I sure felt it.

Of course, there were the literal costs, too. By this time, I had gotten onto Medicare due to my earlier Social Security disability. That turned out to be a godsend overall - Medicare provided a wonderful sense of security after the insurance anxieties of the previous few years. Even so, I still had to pay monthly premiums for it, just like any insurance. Furthermore, Medicare only covered 80% of my medical bills. So every one of those 142 visits resulted in an additional co-pay or uncovered charge. Thanks to Medicare's aggressive price negotiating, most of the individual charges weren't that huge. But they sure started piling up. During those two years, our out-of-pocket medical expenditures (including insurance premiums) totaled $40,017.

Just as burdensome as the money itself, maybe even more so, was the perpetual stack of bills on my desk. For some reason, I found the constant check writing and envelope stamping and expense tracking growing ever more stressful. Maybe it's because of my compulsive nature - I always worry about staying on top of the details and getting everything done right and on time. I guess that's not a bad thing, but it sure creates anxiety and takes up mental energy. More opportunity costs there.

As I reflect back on that period, I realize that all the worries about expenses and bills and paperwork somehow compounded my physical struggles, and vice versa. It all snowballed into an increasingly stressful burden. When I think of the countless other Americans going through similar challenges - in many cases far worse than ours - I think it all weighs down our whole national spirit. Every time I talk about this to folks from Canada or Australia or the northern European countries, they scratch their heads in bemusement. They just don't feel the same stress – healthcare anxieties don't even come on their radar. I wonder if that's why Canadians seem so relaxed and pleasant (except at hockey games).

Speaking of anxieties, I noticed a similar trend with our constant home rehab projects. The expenses were piling up. Some of these were large investments in our property's long-term value, which we were willing to make. But in a quiet, stealthy way, the little expenditures starting accumulating, too: a gallon of paint here and there, lumber for shelves, ceiling panels for the basement, mulch for a planting bed, a new chain for the chainsaw, and so forth.

Just as with the medical bills, the burden was much more than financial. I was constantly thinking of unfinished chores, what comes next, what to add to the perpetual list for my next run to Home Depot. Worrying, too, about drafty windows, and rotting siding, and over-grown gardens, and freezing pipes, and accumulating ice, and mice infesting our basement ceiling, and on and on. My mind was always churning trying to stay on top of it all. Intertwine all that with my physical difficulties keeping up with the chores themselves, and our big home rehab project - while rewarding in so many ways - was weighing me down.

Isn't it an interesting paradox how sometimes you can become almost a victim of your own strengths? I'm usually a methodical, meticulous perfectionist. I'm always worrying about every detail, analyzing every decision, trying to get everything right, figuring out the next steps, always thinking ahead to prevent any stress. Ironically, that often creates a stress of its own. Sometimes I drive myself crazy!

Similarly, Mary Ann has strengths of her own. At work, she's creative, passionate, and driven – an absolutely tenacious competitor. Give her good products to sell, some pay incentives, and a supportive back-office, then set her loose, and she's a high-powered engine of growth. The flip side of that is she doesn't take well to being boxed-in and second-guessed, or held back by the slow pace that companies sometimes settle (or stagnate) into.

And that's exactly what was happening with her job. After having stabilized things at her company's US division, she was now pouring her heart and soul (and 12-14 hours per day) into the pursuit of sales. Even so, the company was going stale. The spirit of innovation, the new product development, the commitment to growth, and yes, the money – the things that motivate her – had all stalled. Her pay, which in great part was based on commissions and bonuses, actually started declining.

Meanwhile, my corporate training was sputtering along. The burden of being the primary breadwinner was weighing heavily on Mary Ann's shoulders. Now I don't want to exaggerate the severity of our financial challenges – compared to so many Americans struggling after the recession, we were still relatively OK. But our declining cash flow and the accumulating expenses were always on our mind, and we could sure use some extra income. So Mary Ann took things into her own hands in a move that just blew me away.

A big new department store was opening up at the Portland Mall, with all sorts of hiring hoopla. Mary Ann saw one of their ads for part-time sales help. Their shoe department in particular appeared to have a lucrative commission structure. Well if you know anything about Mary Ann, she sure loves shoes! She also loves selling, especially when there are commissions to be made. The store allowed her some flexibility around her travel schedule, so she took the job. Can you imagine, a woman with the title of "Vice President" in her day job was working nights at a shoe store!

Well she plunged right in with her typical enthusiasm, working at about twice the pace of everyone else. I went in to visit a few times - I even bought a pair of Skechers for myself. I was amazed, but not surprised, to see Mary Ann hustling from customer to customer, carrying shoe boxes to and fro, kneeling, engaging, connecting – always with personality and a smile. The customers loved her. Managers, too. She was selling the doors off the place. Where in the world did she get that passion, that energy? I was in awe.

Mary Ann's stint in the shoe store hit me in other ways, too, like a wake-up call. Here she was, working long days in her regular job, then hustling off to the shoe store in the evening to bring in some extra cash - and what was I doing to help? Not much. I realized (once again) that I'd been just drifting along, hitching my wagon to a single, often-sporadic source of work, not taking enough initiative to seek out or develop other things on my own. Sure, I wasn't feeling that great, and what little energy I had I was devoting to our house chores. But could those be rationalizations, even excuses? I decided to stretch myself and look for a way to pitch in more. Realistically, I didn't have the stamina for a full-time job – that wasn't an excuse, that was reality. But maybe I could handle a part-time gig. I decided to give it a shot, and the perfect can't-miss place was right down the street.

I think most anyone who knows me would agree that I'm sort of an LL Bean type of guy. The clothes, the gear, the outdoorsy lifestyle, etc. I've long admired Bean for their customer service, high quality (often USA-made) products, environmental policies, and overall vibe. In fact, years ago I came very close to landing a good corporate training job there. (As I recall, that little invisible hand I wrote about earlier held me back.) Now they were hiring a ton of part-time workers for their pre-Christmas rush, so I figured this would be a perfect opportunity to get my foot in the door. A slam dunk. I also knew it would make Mary Ann happy and maybe even a bit proud. I felt suddenly psyched.

So I put on a blue Oxford button-down shirt, crisply pressed Dockers, and of course a pair of nice leather Bean boat shoes. I strode into the HR office ready to knock it out of the park. The interviewer and I started chatting. We hit it off well. My answers to her questions rolled out smoothly. I asked a few good ones of my own. I was in my element, and I was nailing it.

Then the interviewer explained that there might be some clerical aspects to the job, so she asked me to do a few tasks on the computer. The keyboard and monitor were a few feet apart. I leaned over to get a closer look at the monitor. My eyes were irritated, so I asked if I could use my reading glasses. I fumbled around for them in my shirt pocket. She asked me to enter some information from a sheet of paper. I leaned over to take a look. I'm not a touch typist – I have to see the keys. So I hunched back over the keyboard. Suddenly my hands started cramping. I felt awkward and self-conscious hunting for the keys and slowly pecking away with my contorted fingers. I wondered if I was making mistakes - I couldn't tell because I had a hard time seeing the monitor. I felt myself getting tense, even a bit short of breath. Then the kicker: As I leaned back toward the monitor, my hamstring cramped up. I tried to stifle a groan and hide the pain, but I'm sure she saw the grimace on my face. "Sorry, just a little cramp," I lied.

As we wrapped up the interview, she said something about their scheduling needs not meshing with my work travel, so they were going to take a pass on hiring me for now. She suggested I stay in touch. As I walked out (actually limped out), I knew exactly what that meant.

I've had a lot of "jolts" during my cancer journey - those moments when reality hits you like a brick. The first was way back at the beginning when I noticed that hospice brochure in Dr. Diener's waiting room, and a whole string of them followed from there. Well, the jolt from that LL Bean interview was right up there with the best of them. It was more humbling than the lady helping me put my luggage in the overhead bin. More discouraging than walking my bike up a hill or quitting the ski slopes after a couple disastrous runs. And, in its own way, more graphic and jarring than seeing my bloody ear with a chunk missing. In typical fashion, I brushed it off with some light-hearted comment. But on the inside, I felt stunned and disheartened - and maybe even a bit scared.

Where do you find the line between the things you can fight back from, and the things you have to accept as the new reality? That in itself is a part of that constant mental toggling you go through.

Meanwhile, Mary Ann kept working her tail off at the shoe store, motivated by her continued sales success, and fascinated by this glimpse into the world of hourly retail work. She came home each night with all sorts of stories about her co-workers. What an interesting mix: young twenty-somethings just starting out, empty nesters, immigrants, former professionals, even a college athletic coach. They probably wondered about her, too.

Anyway, after a couple months of killer sales, Mary Ann noticed the commissions she was expecting were not showing up in her paycheck. She asked around, and only then did she learn that the hiring discussions had glossed over some "fine print" in the compensation policy. Her commissions would actually turn out to be miniscule. She felt misled. Soon afterward, upper management started coming out with all sorts of silly edicts, including one that prohibited employees from drinking water during their shift! Can you believe that? Who comes up with this stuff? Well these things took the wind out of Mary Ann's sails (pun intended), and she soon left. Apparently, most of the other talent did, too.

We were back to just scraping along. The bills and chores kept piling up. The physical and mental toll kept pulling me down. The burdens on Mary Ann increased. And my symptoms kept getting worse...

So I hope you see what I meant by the phrase "entangled tentacles." My physical problems intertwined with so many other aspects of our life, and vice versa. I was racked with disappointment and self-doubt. Guilt about my meager contributions to our finances. Exhaustion trying to keep up with the house chores. Mental clutter, worries – and deep below the surface, even fears about whether this downturn would be a long decline to the end. I could also feel Mary Ann's stress, which weighed me down further. It all compounded into a negative type of synergy.

It was so disheartening to have climbed back so far in my post-transplant recovery, and now this. In many ways, this setback was a tougher period than the transplant itself and its immediate aftermath. At least then, I was on a path forward. But here there was no path, no predictability, no certainty about anything.

I kept plugging away as best I could. I tried to keep up a positive face, to keep looking on the bright side, finding the silver linings and humor and all that. I don't think I ever took my frustrations out on Mary Ann – at least not directly. But there were plenty of times when I'd be curled up on the couch with disappointment and frustration churning through my mind, my body seized by cramps or contortions or aches or stomach pain or burning eyes or total utter fatigue - or any combination thereof - and sometimes I'd let a little self-pity bubble out. Sometimes a plea for sympathy, or a gripe about the unfairness of it all. Sometimes an out-loud prayer to God just asking for a break. At least that's what I thought I was saying. Mary Ann later confided that she occasionally heard me say something much darker...

Part 10

CLIMBING BACK AGAIN

$\mathcal{P}$endulum swings can take many forms.

One morning, I was out in California just about to begin a workshop. I noticed a voicemail message from Mary Ann on my phone, so I grabbed it. You know how you can instantly tell when something's wrong by the first syllable in one's voice? Well I sure could: "There's... there's... been an explosion... The house next to ours is gone... We have lots of damage... The cats are OK – I got 'em quarantined in the bedroom... I'm walking into the living room now, and... oh my god, there's glass everywhere and stuff knocked over..."

There had been a propane leak in the house next door. It exploded into smithereens, leaving nothing but the concrete foundation. The fellow living there was killed. Apparently the blast was heard 15 miles away. Only 80 yards away, our house suffered significant damage: windows blown in, siding ripped off, cracks in the chimney, some structural damage to the studs, and much more. When I got back home, my first impression was of a war zone, as if our house had been bombed. Come to think of it, it had. I just shook my head in disbelief. Here we go again - one more challenge to deal with.

What was that I was saying earlier about jolts? Well, sometimes a jolt can be a good thing - it can push the pendulum in a positive direction. And you know what? Despite the unfortunate loss of life next

223

door and many months of inconvenience to us, that's exactly what ended up happening with the explosion. It helped propel us forward, in many ways.

A great part of that was due to my brothers. They're both private insurance adjusters - they help businesses and homeowners file claims for major losses. My brother Eric in particular guided us through the complex process of preparing a comprehensive claim and negotiating with the insurance company. Without his help, we probably would have settled for the insurance company's initial low-ball offer. He ended up getting us a much better settlement. That allowed us to get the damage repaired fully, and the house fixed up better than ever.

An additional side benefit: getting a real-life glimpse into the professional expertise of a family member in full work mode. I think we often take each other's professional skills for granted.

The repairs took many months. Our house was pretty much torn apart all over. There were construction workers all over the place – inside, outside, up on the roof. Early one morning we were startled awake by a guy on a ladder prying off the remains of our bedroom window! It may have been a bit disruptive, but overall it was actually fascinating and even fun. We kept the crew well supplied with drinks and snacks. They particularly loved Mary Ann's home-baked cookies. Near the end of the work day, I'd sometimes sneak a beer or two into their pick-up cabs. It was so cool to get to know the guys, hear their stories, and get to appreciate *their* professional skills – they were amazing carpenters.

With cold weather closing in, it was a race to finish up the repairs and finally get the exterior of the house repainted. Mary Ann and I had spent weeks experimenting with different color samples – this would be our chance to get rid of the dreary old brownish-rust color, and unleash the house's underlying character. We carefully chose a custom grey for the siding, soft white for the trim, black for the shutters, and a deep red for the garage and shed doors. We asked the painters to do the front side last. They finished it while we were away. I'll always remember the thrill of coming home and pulling into the driveway – our jaws dropped. What a transformation! It was like one of those home makeover shows on TV. The rough had been polished off the diamond, and now it glistened.

That explosion ultimately helped moved us forward. It accelerated what probably would have been years of puttering and tinkering into a quick surge. It lifted a burden off us, especially me. It added value (and curb appeal) to our property. It gave us the uplifting satisfaction of seeing a vision realized. Coupled with the great help we received from so many others, it showed that you can recover, repair, and rebuild better than ever. I'd like to think there was some symbolism there.

Another type of explosion also helped move us forward, though in a totally different way. It was an absolutely beautiful day. Mary Ann was all packed and ready for her trip to China later that afternoon. She really wanted to get in a bike ride before being cooped up on planes for so long. I prepared the bikes as usual, and got ready to tag along. As we discussed our route, I could sense a little something going on.

We started riding. As usual those days, I soon fell behind. A couple miles down the road, she was waiting for me at a stop sign. We started again. Soon we came to a big hill. Again, she surged ahead. I struggled badly on the hill, and I had to get off and walk part of the way. By the time I reached her at the top, I was shot. I said I had to turn back. I encouraged Mary Ann to keep going, but she abruptly turned around, and we both headed back home. Soon she was way ahead out of sight.

When I finally made it back home, I could tell she was fuming. I apologized for my slow pace. She exploded. I don't remember all the words, but at the end she screamed out, "I just wanted to get in a good ride, and you were holding me back! Your disease is holding me back!" It felt like a dagger went through me. I dissolved in sobs...

...It didn't take long for both of us to recover our composure. It was like after a violent thunderstorm passes, when the air suddenly seems clear and calm. We had a good talk. That was the first time in the seven plus years since my initial diagnosis that she'd said anything even remotely like that. I cut her some slack - imagine the stress *she'd* kept bottled up all this time. It was good to let it out.

225

And the thing is, she had a point. I knew she had a limited amount of time to get in a good ride, and I knew I wouldn't be able to keep up. So why did I automatically just glom onto her? That was a good wake-up call, a reminder that we all need a little space of our own from time to time. A reminder of a vital lesson to all cancer patients and survivors: It's not always about *you* - it's also about the caregiver, the partner.

Like peeling away the layers of an onion, I kept thinking about this incident at an even deeper level. I realized that at its core, Mary Ann's explosion probably had little to do with the bike ride itself. That was just the trigger. Imagine the accumulated stress she'd kept pent up for all those years; imagine all the sacrifices she'd made, dreams she'd put on hold; imagine how it felt seeing her once-strong husband no longer in the lead, struggling, deteriorating, maybe even slipping away. All that was the fuel. Why hadn't I realized this before?

From the pain of that incident came a lesson on one of the most valuable ingredients of all, not just for cancer couples, but for any relationship: empathy. Not just the superficial kind. Empathy with a capital E. The kind that runs deep, way below the outer layers of the onion.

In a strange and surprising way, I somehow felt better after our bike ride blow-up. I think Mary Ann did, too.

***

Jolts and explosions are one thing, but sometimes little nudges help push things along, too. Mary Ann has given me some great gifts over the years. Once I told her that I regretted never learning to play a musical instrument. She said it's never too late. Next thing I knew, she contacted a friend in the music business, and surprised me with a beautiful guitar. I was blown away. I was just starting to get the hang of playing it when my GVH intensified and my fingers stopped working. I dream of picking it up again someday. Another time, she came back from northern India with a surprise gift: a local artist's painting of Mt. Everest. That was such a sweet, touching gesture. I look up at that painting in my office every day.

And during this tough stretch, when she could tell I was feeling down and in a bit of a rut, she gave me one of the most powerful gifts of all: Just a little scrap of paper she'd torn out somewhere containing a quote from William Faulkner. (We've always had friendly debates about Faulkner. She loves him - I can never get my head around his writing style.) Anyway, the quote was about stretching - reaching for things just beyond your grasp. It stirred something in me. On one level, it was a little nudge to keep striving and growing. More deeply, it was also a gentle reminder never to let my cancer or its after-effects be a crutch for lethargy. Just as with the Mt. Everest painting, I look at that scrap of paper every day.

I gave *her* a little nudge during this time, too. I've already described how Mary Ann was in a rut of her own at her job. Well, we started picking up hints that there might be a chance to return to the company she'd spent most of career with before – the place she'd built her greatest success. They'd gone through a long series of organizational changes and purges, and it now appeared that one of their main product lines was ripe for rejuvenation – a product line right in Mary Ann's wheelhouse. I kept nudging her to give them a call. No, come to think of it, it was stronger than nudging - outright nagging was more like it.

Finally she made the call, and guess what? That opened the door, and they soon welcomed her back. It was almost like coming home after a long wayward odyssey. It reinvigorated her. Her passion was back. And let's not kid ourselves – the money helped a lot, too! We were moving ahead again.

One more thing propelled us on our climb back. It started with a look in the mirror and a big realization. Mary Ann was traveling extensively in her new job, often with long trips overseas. I had to face the music that my strength and stamina weren't what they used to be. Though we'd made great strides with our house and it now looked beautiful, it would certainly require ongoing upkeep inside and out. Knowing me, I'd probably be tinkering and puttering away forever. We realized that maybe a big house and yard wasn't for us at this stage in our lives. So, a few years after we'd moved down from the mountains to be closer to civilization, it was time to think about another swing of the pendulum.

Though we lived within easy striking distance of downtown Portland, it was still a drive. In fact, we had to drive most everywhere. What about a more urban, drive-less-walk-more lifestyle? A place where we wouldn't be so beholden to constant house and yard chores? A place that would free us (especially me) for other pursuits? After all, that was becoming a huge trend. From young entrepreneurs to baby boomer empty-nesters, folks everywhere were migrating back into the cities. My brother Eric and sister-in-law Marcia moved away from the suburbs and into the heart of Boston as soon as their kids left the house, and they loved it. Also my mother had long been hinting that we'd be happy in a more urban setting.

And one more insight hit me about this, a huge one: That's where Mary Ann's heart was, too! I realized that she'd never been much for house maintenance and especially yard work. (Just ask her parents sometime about all the ways she used to finagle herself out of doing yard chores when she was a kid – apparently, she'd feign illness or injury, or sneak off and hide behind a bush with a book in hand!) As much as we both made fun of her "urban hipster" longings, that was actually more of her true calling. After all, she'd been living in a funky loft in the cool part of Old Montreal when I lured her away to the remote New Hampshire woods.

It dawned on me that I hadn't really been listening to her as well as I could have. Listening fully, deeply, like with a capital L. I guess I'd been imposing my own outdoorsy-handyman-cut-your-own-firewood type of lifestyle on us. Sometimes I even joked that I wanted to go "live off the grid" somewhere! Even though this was purely self-mocking humor, at some level it must have terrified her. All humor aside, I realized that in my own easy-going-let's-all-get-along manner, I can be very set in my ways sometimes.

Even though I just mentioned cities, I don't think I would ever want to live in a big one like New York, or even smaller Boston. But little Portland was a good compromise – everything you'd want in a city, but livable, outdoorsy, and close to nature. The latter were still important to me – part of my own "true calling" if you will. We started poking around downtown Portland, exploring neighborhoods, checking out different locations and types of residences. It was like trying on clothes at the store, getting a sense of what fits and feels best.

One day we were driving around just beyond the edge of the bustling downtown. It seemed to be an area in transition, a mix of empty lots, abandoned old buildings, a few new ones, bordered by a real brick-sidewalk neighborhood on one side and a waterfront park on the other. Nearby were coffee shops, bakeries, and small European style produce markets. It seemed everyone was walking a dog. You could hear sea gulls from the nearby harbor, and catch glimpses of tugboats going by.

We drove past an empty lot, overgrown with weeds and strewn with trash. There was a chain link fence all around, which looked as if it had been put up recently. We noticed a sign on the fence showing a new building planned for the site – a small residential building. I jammed on the brakes. "What a location," I exclaimed. "This is the place! It couldn't be more perfect!" I rolled down the passenger window. Mary Ann snapped a picture of the sign. We raced back home, did some quick Internet research, and called the number on the sign. The next morning, we zipped back down, asked a few questions, and wrote a deposit check on the spot. How's that for a "time-to-do-this" decision?

Instantly, everything changed. It felt as if a huge weight had been lifted off our shoulders: the burden of constantly tending to, and worrying about, our house and yard. A new, more urban lifestyle beckoned.

We playfully started fantasizing about our life to come. We pictured ourselves strolling across the street to a funky sidewalk cafe, hanging out with laptops open, sipping our exotic coffee concoctions, petting the dogs that stop by our table (and sneaking them pieces of our muffins); meandering along the harbor watching the tugboats; stopping at a farmers' market to pick up some organic produce and artisanal cheese (while of course making fun of the word "artisanal"); walking to galleries and theaters and live music shows. Mary Ann even kidded that she'd get a tattoo. (I sure as hell hope she was kidding.) We were instantly energized by this impending change in our world - or to put it into classic Maine-speak, wicked psyched!

And believe it or not, I soon started feeling better. No, not perfect - this isn't a fairy tale - but definitely a bit lighter, less entangled, more invigorated. There could have been any number of reasons: The easing of our house maintenance burdens, excitement toward our new life ahead, Dr. Soiffer's tweaks to my medications, my GVH disease subsiding, maybe some random good luck, and maybe a combination of them all.

But I also think something bigger was going on. I think much of this upturn had to do with the power of accepting new realities, shedding old burdens, evolving out of ruts, creating new visions, even listening to your partner...

The present day

A little disclosure here. The chronology of our story has now slipped past the timing in the title. The events I just described took place in year seven, and by the time I get this all polished and wrapped up, it'll be well into year eight. You know me: slow and methodical – often agonizingly so! Anyway, I'm going to stick with my original title, mainly because it's short and snappy. But whatever the year count, by far the most important words in the title are the last two.

So let me briefly bring you up to the present day. Things have happened fast. When we made the deal for the new condo, we knew it would take at least a year for the building to be completed, so we had lots of time to prepare our house for sale. It didn't need much more work – we had gotten it to the point where it practically staged itself (thanks in great part to my mother's decorating help). One day we were chatting with a real estate agent about the best long-term sales strategy, and we decided we'd put it on the market several months down the road. As we wrapped up the conversation, I tossed in a quick comment something to the effect of, "If you run across an interested buyer in the meantime, let us know."

Well be careful what you ask for. The very next day, she brought over a buyer, and the day after that we had a deal. Full asking price, all cash, no contingencies, and they wanted to close in a month. Whoa, time to move fast! This was going to be a huge downsizing. We put most of our furniture for sale on Craigslist. Buyers soon started trooping through our house. We scurried around and found an apartment to move into. I lugged carloads of stuff to Goodwill. More carloads to our local transfer station (or as everyone actually called it, the dump). I'd been feeling pretty good anyway, but this surge of adrenaline or whatever it was kicked me into an even higher gear. I hadn't felt this energized in years. It was like an invisible hand lifting me, keeping me going, holding me up... and I didn't fall back down. Sisyphus was nowhere to be seen.

We took a chance by holding a rare January garage sale. Fortunately, the weather cooperated, and a ton of people showed up. We hustled around our garage around like crazy, selling things left and right. Sort of reminded me of Mary Ann at the shoe store. Items were flying out as quickly as we could collect the money. It was a blast. Within a couple hours, we were almost totally cleaned out. Afterward, we went back into the warmth of the house, dumped our thick wads of cash onto the table, gave each other a high-five, and poured the first of several drinks.

A little side story from the garage sale: One guy came up to me ready to pay for a load of rakes, shovels, gardening supplies, clippers, and other tools, all piled into our wheelbarrow. Suddenly he noticed my chainsaw over in the corner – my beloved trusty Stihl companion for so many years. He asked, "How much do you want for that chainsaw?" I took a breath, thought for a couple seconds, and said "Take it!"

We're now living in a temporary apartment while our new place is under construction. Life is much simpler. We don't miss all our stuff. (George Carlin was sure right on target with his classic "stuff" routine years ago.) Our apartment is near the Portland airport, and we often take evening strolls over to the edge of the runway. As often as Mary Ann and I each fly for our work, for some reason we still get a childish thrill watching the planes take off and land. There's something so majestic about it. Of course, that often gets us bantering with faux pilot talk: "Looks like the 18:25 UAL from IAD, on approach from the east." "Roger that. Visual contact established." "What's your vector, Victor," and so on. After all these years, we still make each other laugh.

And we still enrich each other's minds. Well, maybe I shouldn't speak for Mary Ann's mind, but she sure keeps enriching *mine*. She continues to devour books and articles at a staggering pace – she constantly scours websites and social media for all sorts of fascinating articles. Sometimes she drives me crazy the way she always has a book or her laptop open, or even both! But I love it – she shares the gist of what she's reading, like my own personalized Reader's Digest service. I learn things. We have stimulating conversations. And I'd like to think I teach her a few things now and then, too.

All this reminds me of a little side story Mary Ann told me only recently about her elementary school days. It speaks volumes. Many years ago, she got in big trouble for forging a pass to get out of study hall. But it wasn't the usual thing kids do, like to sneak out and goof off somewhere. No, she had finished all her assignments, she had nothing to read, and she was bored. So she forged a pass to go to the library, of all places, so she could read! I wonder how the principal handled that. On the surface, he probably gave her a stern, intimidating lecture about the importance of honesty and all that. But I bet on the inside, he was quietly chuckling. In any case, I'm glad that little bookworm grew up to become my wife.

On the work front these days, Mary Ann is working her tail off, as usual. Traveling all over the world, opening new markets in all sorts of places. Right now as I type this, she's on her way to Accra, Ghana. How's that for a new market? I don't know how she keeps up such a pace, but I'm thankful she does – she's winning plenty of bread. Just as important, she's challenged and engaged and involved. You know what all that adds up to: The passion is back. And passion can be contagious.

As for me, my regular workshop volume has picked up, and I'm contributing my fair share to our revenue these days. I've also got a few new things cooking on the side - I hope to be opening some "new markets" of my own soon. Once I finish up this book, I'll plunge in further. Can't wait.

Our new condo is coming along. We've selected the finishes and tiles and appliances and all that. Mary Ann and Nancy have been picking out furniture and lamps. It's going to be a stylish place, sort of chic and contemporary – a whole new decor for us. I'm fine with that – a little change is healthy. Every chance we get, we check out the construction. It's been exciting to watch that overgrown vacant lot slowly transform into a beautiful new building, with ocean views in one direction and a funky neighborhood in the other. Each time we stop by, we pinch ourselves that this is actually going to be our new home, and our new world.

Nancy's feeling good – she's now 88. She's fought her way back from her leg injury several years ago, plus a more recent back injury, and she's spry as ever. Sharp as ever, too. She's been spending hours online searching for furniture and fixtures to give our new place just the right touch of style. I think she's even more psyched than we are. I love the way Nancy and Mary Ann stay connected by exchanging emails with all their furnishing ideas – even when Mary Ann's on another continent! I can't wait for the three of us to walk in to the new place together and see our vision brought to life.

I continue to feel better overall, slowly climbing back from my physical downturn of the last few years. No, it's not like some sudden miracle – everything's still a struggle, and the symptoms continue. My dry eyes in particular continue to be a problem. But at least I've regained enough energy and strength to take some small steps forward.

One example: A few months ago, Mary Ann and I decided to do some spring skiing before another ski season slipped away. We headed up to Sunday River – the first time we'd gone to a full-size ski area together in several years. I was quietly apprehensive about how I'd feel – my previous few attempts to ski had not gone well. We rode the lift to the top. The view was beautiful. The snow was good. Mary Ann started down first. She skis the way she does most everything - she just goes and goes.

I took a deep breath and pushed off after her. I made a few cautious turns. They felt OK. A few more, a bit faster. Still feeling fine – breathing OK and no cramps or muscle burn. Faster still, longer turns, deeper carves. Suddenly, long-dormant technique come back to life and took hold of me. I let loose, feeling that old familiar rush of G's on each turn. I swooped my way down and carved a big arc past Mary Ann - I'm not sure if she heard me whooping and singing as I went by. Finally I had to stop for a breather. I turned around and watched her come down. She still has some lingering pain from her injuries, but as she glided toward me, all I saw was a smile. We kept going like that, run after run.

The après-ski vibes out on the deck that day were especially sweet. The reggae was thumping, the beer tasted great, and we even ran into some old instructor pals from Bretton Woods. Life doesn't get much better than sharing a great day on the slopes with your wife and friends.

It's now summer, and on the bike I've been feeling stronger, too. I can make it up the hills these days without stopping. Mary Ann usually doesn't have to wait too long for me at the top, if at all. We've done a few 50 mile rides together, and I can hold my own keeping up with her most of the way. I even surged past her going up a hill the other day! And she wasn't letting me - she'd never do that.

Beyond the sports activities, I've found myself a bit more "functional" going about the basic tasks of daily life. It's subtle. You notice the little things, like being able to reach down and pick things up off the floor, or hoisting your luggage into the overhead bin, or going a whole day without having to take a nap, or taking a walk and deciding to take the long loop back home.

At the same time, the various symptoms and side effects keep tugging at you – totally random and unpredictable, usually mere nuisances, occasionally frustrations, and always reminders - reminding you every day that you're never "over it."

I still have my regular visits with Dr. Soiffer down at Dana Farber every few months. He reviews my symptoms, pokes and prods a little, checks and interprets my lab numbers, tweaks meds when necessary, and always frames things in the big picture perspective. Nancy often comes with me – they like to chat about local Boston gossip. It's been great to develop such a human connection with the guy who helped save my life.

An amazing thing happened recently at one of my appointments with Soiffer. He sometimes has to multi-task between different patients, and I was waiting in the exam room while he was meeting with someone else. I was feeling pretty good that day. Suddenly he popped his head into the room and said, "Hey Peter, can you come out here? There's someone I'd like you to meet." He walked me down the hall into another exam room. There sat a couple who appeared to be in their late 40's. I noticed their hands were clasped together, and they had that look in their eyes. I could tell immediately what it meant. Soiffer introduced us. Yes, it turned out the guy was facing a bone marrow transplant, and they were having "the conversation." They were avid skiers. Soiffer made a point of telling them that I had returned to being a ski instructor after my transplant. We chatted for a while about New England ski areas, even a few of our favorite runs. I offered them my contact information, and invited them to stay in touch. As I left, all I could think of to say was, "Let's take a run together one of these days."

What a classy move by Dr. Soiffer. I remembered years ago when Mary Ann and I were in the same boat, and he introduced us to one of his recent transplant patients. That made a huge impression on me, just seeing and chatting with a real live transplant survivor in front of me. I hoped that in some small way, my visit with that couple had a similar effect.

————— ❧ —————

And that's the spirit in which I'd like to bring this story into its home stretch. I'm not quite sure what to call it – lots of phrases come to mind: Completing the cycle? Giving something back? Paying it forward? Lending a helping hand? Whatever you call it, it's all about trying to do a little something to share our experiences to help others.

It's been wonderful to see all the various steps our friends and relatives have taken over the years, and continue to take to this day. Whether registering to be potential donors, or spreading the word to others, or participating in fund-raising walks, or just making direct monetary contributions for cancer research, it's all good.

I particularly love it when young people take actions. For example, our niece Julia registered as a donor soon after she turned 18, and not long after that she came close to being the final selection to donate to a transplant patient in need. Very cool. When our nephew Sam was in high school, his soccer team competed each year in a "Kicks for Cancer" fund-raising soccer tournament. The players got special pink uniforms embroidered with their choice of name. Sam chose to wear my family nickname "Woofus" on his jersey, which was quite an honor. (Don't ask about that nickname.)

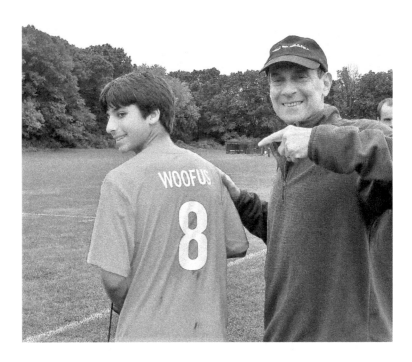

Sam's in college now, and soon he'll be going to Israel on one of those birthright tours for US students. Among many other things, he's going to participate in a Gift of Life presentation and donor registration. In Israel, of all places - how appropriate is that?

I've been making appearances at health fairs and donor drives. Sometimes I just stand there, hoping to give a human face to the signs and posters. Often I'll chat with passersby, answering their questions and, at the right time, sharing bits of my own story. I hope that seeing and talking with a real live transplant survivor might help motivate people to take action steps of their own, whatever form they make take.

Last year, Mary Ann and I gave a talk and showed some slides at our local cancer center. It was great to work together - after all, this was the story of *both* of us. In fact, that was one of the main themes of our presentation: Cancer journeys are a team effort. A few weeks ago, I went back to the same cancer center to listen to another presentation on blood cancer research. A woman in the audience recognized me. She told me she'd recently been through a transplant of her own, and our talk had been very helpful to her and her husband. She looked great. Wow...

A few months ago I was out in Los Angeles for a corporate workshop, and I looked up my donor Eric Rothman. He's doing great. He's landed a sports broadcasting gig for the Los Angeles Lakers' D-League basketball team. Once in a while he calls a game on ESPN. Even more exciting news - he's engaged! We met for dinner, and I met his fiancé. It was a warm, wonderful evening. I can't really put it into words, but there was something special about seeing the guy who helped renew my life now embarking on this exciting new chapter of his own.

One of the biggest highlights for me recently was to be the keynote presenter at a big cancer awareness retreat for 500 high school students. I showed slides and shared my story, with the primary goal to motivate them to register as potential bone marrow donors. My donor Eric wrote a touching piece for the occasion, which I read aloud to the group. I could tell the kids were right there with me. Several of the chaperones said they'd never seen all 500 so quiet and rapt.

Afterwards, lots of students came up and thanked me; many mentioned how cancer had affected their own family members. I was deeply moved. Say what you want about "kids these days," but these kids were amazing. Most gratifying of all was to see so many (18-year-olds) swabbing away at the Gift of Life donor registration table in the back. That event was one of the most enjoyable and rewarding things I've ever done. I hope to have many more evenings like that.

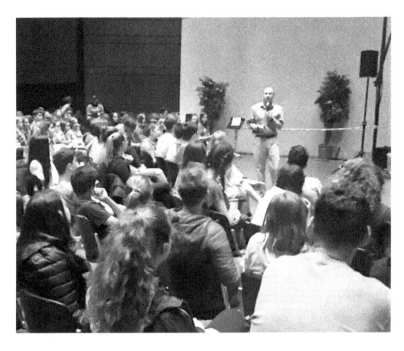

Sometimes I wish I could just package all this up in some way - and then spread it around to all the folks out there who could use a helping hand, or a gentle push, or a glimpse into a real life cancer story. That's the purpose that's been churning inside me, looking to find an outlet. And I guess that's what much of this book has turned out to be – a voice for that purpose. As I said before, purpose is healthy. And I've discovered mine.

Part 11

LESSONS FROM
HINDSIGHT

I hated history way back in high school. All I remember is having to memorize a bunch of dates and kings and battles. It meant
nothing to me. Wow, has that sure changed in recent years! Maybe
it's a natural byproduct of aging, or maybe it's from being married to
a history buff, or most likely a combination of both. In any case, it's
been very gratifying to gain a deeper appreciation of history, and the
wisdom that can come from hindsight.

And I hope to apply some of that here. I'd like to take a look back
over our healthcare journey and share some of the insights that have
crystalized and resonated with Mary Ann and me over the years. Call
them lessons if you want, though we don't mean to lecture or preach
in any way. Consider this section more like a grab-bag; feel free to
reach in and take whatever you find of value.

To put a little structure to the grab-bag, it's divided into two main
sections: The first is geared primarily toward healthcare providers,
though anyone who ever goes to the doctor might find it helpful. It's
called "Doctoring: The good, the bad, and the indifferent."

The second part is written primarily for cancer patients and their
loved ones, though it might also apply to people going through

other health challenges. Providers may find some value in this section as well. It's called "Many medicines besides drugs."

After these two sections, I'll share a few personal reflections. Then I'll bring our story to a close. I really mean it this time. No more false summits. I promise.

Doctoring: The good, the bad, and the indifferent

Mary Ann came up with that title. I like it – it's catchy. But let me reframe it a bit before we get to the specifics. First of all, I'm not even sure if "doctoring" is technically a real word. But I'm going to use it as such, in particular as a term based on a verb – an action word. Because ultimately, it's not a doctor's knowledge or background that counts – it's what he/she actually *does* that makes a difference to patients.

And while we're at it, let's broaden the term "doctoring" to include not just doctors, but nurses, assistants, technicians, administrative staff, and everybody involved in the delivery of health care. They all have a hand in the actions that ultimately affect the patient.

I'll also lump "the indifferent" in with "the bad," and take care of that section first. I'd prefer to end this part with the positives.

Bad doctoring

From what I understand, one of the primary lessons in medical training is "first do no harm." Well I'd like to share a few doctoring traits Mary Ann and I experienced that were harmful, or hurtful, or just left a bad taste with us. It's not my purpose to call out any individuals or institutions specifically. In their own way, I'm sure everyone's just trying to do the best they can. Rather, I'd like to lay out a few things that providers should try to avoid, and patients might want to be on the lookout for.

You might recall that way back near the beginning of this journey, we made our first visit to the first cancer hospital, and it did not go very well. Let me extract some of the specific "doctoring" flaws we noticed in that encounter - things that not only turned us away, but also lost that hospital a huge amount of revenue:

Lack of preparation: Prior to our first visit, we had followed through with everything we were supposed to do ahead of time, as directed. We forwarded my medical records, filled out all the forms, made sure my biopsy slides and labs were sent in, etc. But when we arrived at the hospital, there were all sorts of delays while the staff scrambled around looking for these things. We even ended up having to fill out several forms multiple times. All that confusion and lack of preparation made us wonder how they'd handle the infinitely more complex task of managing my bone marrow transplant.

An unengaging doctor manner: From the moment he first walked in, the lead doctor who would be in charge of my transplant was very unengaging. He barely said hello, made little eye contact, and showed no empathy toward what we were going through. He never referenced the particulars of my case or asked us questions. Instead, he droned on about bone marrow transplants in an aloof, lecturing manner - a lecture, by the way, that rambled and lacked almost any specific substance. We were in completely foreign territory here, so we had no frame of reference about what to expect. Even so, it all felt odd and unsettling – there was just no connection there. That might be fine with simpler, less serious types of doctoring tasks. But with a high-stakes, often stressful condition like cancer, I think interpersonal connection is critical.

Discussing insurance in the exam room: Somewhere in the middle of the doctor's ramble, he suddenly stepped out while the insurance person came in. She asked us lots of questions, and had us fill out a few forms. The doc came back in and resumed his lecture. Then the same thing happened again – more insurance questions and forms. What in the world was going on? At one point, Mary Ann asked her something about whether our transplant would be covered, and she replied "It depends on your insurance." I thought this all seemed a bit awkward, but Mary Ann was totally pissed. Can you imagine how this made her feel? There's certainly a time and place to go over insurance, but never, never in the treatment room.

Vague follow-up plans: To this day, we both still scratch our heads remembering the weird way that meeting wrapped up. I finally managed to ask the doc a question about my supposedly severe diagnosis, something about what comes next. His only answer was "Let's wait and see what happens over the next six months." And then the kicker: He said if they forget to contact us to set up that visit, to call back and remind them. Imagine how that felt. It plunged us into that awful limbo of uncertainty, which in many ways is even more stressful than the cancer itself. Never let a cancer patient leave an appointment without a clear sense of what comes next.

That whole visit was like a case study in how *not* to manage the intake of a cancer patient. It made us wonder if they didn't feel confident they could handle my case, or if they didn't want to take it at all. That may very well be the case in some situations, but if so, providers shouldn't dance around it with fuzzy vagueness. Just come out and say so directly. More on that topic later.

Once we found our way into the capable hands of Dana Farber Cancer Institute, most of my doctoring encounters ended up being positive ones. However, Mary Ann's orthopedic odyssey was a different story. She never found a single, central, trusted medical adviser. Instead, we bounced from doctor to doctor, encountering a mixed bag of experiences along the way. Here are some that fall into the "bad doctoring" category:

Overconfidence and false promises: The night Mary Ann first broke her ankle, the Emergency Room staff called in an orthopedic surgeon to take a look at it; he was filling in that weekend as the hospital's "visiting" orthopedist. When he first looked at the X-rays, he told us she'd suffered a pretty bad break. We asked if he could fix it, and he snapped back almost with a huff that "any board-certified surgeon" could handle the repair. It was late, we were exhausted, and we had no idea what else to do, so we consented to have him perform the surgery. He did it that night, and flew home the next morning. Well that turned out to be a big mistake on our part. He did a poor job. It launched Mary Ann into a long, difficult orthopedic nightmare. The lessons? Beware of overconfident bravado and false promises, and don't make hasty decisions in a stressful atmosphere.

Saying "You should have:" Mary Ann suffered through excruciating pain that night. The night nurse didn't teach her how to use the morphine pump properly. Apparently, the nurse just ran through a quick verbal overview, and never checked to make sure Mary Ann (who was still groggy from anesthesia) could actually perform the task. Her pleas for pain relief during the night were ignored. The next morning, as the nurse was wrapping up her shift, she stopped in and discovered what Mary Ann had been doing wrong with the pump all night. Instead of apologizing or showing some empathy, the nurse rudely snapped at her something to the effect of "You should have..." and so on. I've always found virtually all nurses to be wonderful, but that one sure had ineffective teaching skills and a horrible bedside manner. Never, never say "You should have..." to a patient.

Failure to acknowledge limitations: Before long, it was clear that Mary Ann's ankle had not been repaired properly, and she'd need a second surgery. We eventually found our way into the hands of another orthopedist – maybe "stumbled our way" is the better description. This doctor had quite the opposite manner as the first guy – he seemed sort of lackadaisical about wanting to fix her ankle. We almost had to coax him into doing the surgery. Afterwards, the ankle never felt right to Mary Ann, and her foot started looking increasingly disfigured. Even so, the doc discharged her, almost as if he didn't want to have ownership of her problem anymore. As it turned out, this surgery had also been done poorly, leading to many more months of pain for Mary Ann and frustration for both of us. In hindsight, it was partially our mistake again – we should have read the signals about his lack of confidence, and made a better decision. But the doc sure could have been more honest and direct with us about his limitations – he knew that surgery was over his head.

243

Indifference and dismissiveness: Not long after her fall, Mary Ann started feeling increasing pain in her knee. Through some referrals, we made our way to a knee specialist down in Boston – a three-hour drive. His assistants did some preliminary checks on Mary Ann's knee, and entered some notes. Then the doctor swooped in. He glanced at the notes, then felt around her knee for about twenty seconds. He asked a quick question or two, but didn't say anything further. Then he abruptly left, asking us to follow up with his assistant. As we were waiting out in the hall to learn the next steps (there wouldn't be any), we overheard him dictating his notes. He sounded rushed and disinterested. The gist was that he was writing her off without any further recommendations. One specific phrase we heard him say was "typical middle-aged woman." That was not only dismissive and rude, but it masked his failure to notice that she had substantial patella damage that would eventually require two more surgeries. He sure never got that work.

I'd like to share a few more observations here. These are not so much from any particular encounter we had, but rather miscellaneous doctoring issues we've noticed in general.

Unrealistic hope: This is a tough one to write about. It comes from something we've heard occasionally from other cancer families. While I certainly value the power of optimism, I think some doctors might take it too far. Or maybe more accurately, they provide hope without framing it in a realistic perspective. Several times we've heard fellow cancer couples clinging to what seemed like unrealistic expectations, almost like a form of denial. Apparently, their doctors never gave them anything except optimism – empty of substance and disembodied from context. It's been tough to bite our tongues and be as encouraging as we can when all the signals pointed otherwise. And it's been heartbreaking to hear their anguish as reality finally sets in. I've mentioned many times my belief that when there's no tangible information to latch onto, the mind tends to fill the blanks in its own way. Whether this leads to unfounded fears or unrealistic expectations, I think neither is in the best interest of patients and their partners.

Feeling rushed: This is more of a general trend we've noticed with some (though not all) of our doctor visits, and I'm sure we're far from alone. After you arrive on time for your appointment, you wait for ages in the waiting room. Then once you finally get to see the doctor, the visit feels rushed. You leave without fully understanding things or getting a chance to ask all your questions. Yes, I know doctors are under constant pressure to increase efficiency and hit productivity targets and all that. Schedules are jammed tight with patients. It sort of reminds me of what's happened with air travel - at least in coach. So I think it's more of a systematic issue with today's healthcare model overall, rather than the fault of the doctors themselves. Can't do much about that here. But I wonder if a little more time with the doctor might lead to better patient outcomes. That would sure make a good research project.

The barrage of drug ads: Please allow me to toss in one more gripe about our healthcare system these days. It's all the drug ads you see on TV! A few years ago, it was sort of funny to see those silly Cialis commercials with the couple in separate bath tubs. But recently these ads have fallen into a repetitive and irritating pattern: "If you think you may be suffering from (insert disease), ask your doctor about (insert drug name)." It particularly bugs me when I see ads for cancer drugs – something's not right with that picture. No disrespect meant to the individual drugs themselves - I probably wouldn't be alive today if it weren't for some powerful ones. It's more the constant marketing barrage directed at consumers. I wrote something earlier about how insurance bills and paperwork are weighing down the spirit of the American public. Well in many ways, I think the constant drumbeat of these drug ads might be doing much the same thing. And don't even get me started about the inflated price of drugs in our country – that's a rant for another time. Anyway, thanks for letting me get that off my chest - I feel better. Especially now that we're turning to the "good doctoring" part.

Good doctoring

If I listed every positive encounter we've had with medical providers over our journey, this book would never end. So instead, I've tried to distill all these experiences into several key attributes of good doctoring. A reminder that these are just our observations and opinions, and other patients may have different views. I hope you find some of these helpful:

Combining kindness with directness: I'll always remember the way Dr. Diener talked me through my first bone marrow biopsy. He explained precisely what he was doing each step of the way, but in a caring, calming tone. Then the way he first broke the news that I had a dangerous form of cancer: Kind, calm, and empathetic, but also straightforward and direct. A great combination - a model for all providers to try to emulate.

Organized intake of new patients: In stark contrast to the first cancer hospital we visited, Dana Farber did everything right when they brought us on board. They were well prepared and decisive at our first visit. I'll always remember the helpful agenda they sent before our first meeting with the transplant team. The meeting itself was smoothly organized – efficient but never rushed. Dr. Soiffer exuded calm confidence. The head nurse walked us through a huge, potentially overwhelming reference binder, having already placed little sticky notes on the most important sections. When we returned later for our hospital orientation, we found the same thing – a well-planned and informative day. The whole process seemed to combine thorough preparation with empathy for the patient and family. And that's pretty much the way my whole transplant went, too.

Keeping the patient informed and involved: Dr. Diener's bone marrow biopsy reminds me of a doctoring trait that I've found helpful: Let the patient know what you're doing, and why. My dentist always does a great job of this while he's working away inside my mouth. My ear surgeons did the same (on my ear, not my mouth). We've found

Emergency Room staffs are great at this, always explaining not only what they're doing, but *why*. I even like it when the technicians taking my vital signs share the readings with me. It's all about keeping the patient informed and involved. I still remember my surgery to install Hickman catheters right after I checked in for my transplant hospitalization. Even though I was semi-conscious from the anesthesia, the team kept explaining what they were doing, asking if I was OK, even cracking a few jokes. Feeling involved like that gave me confidence as I entered my long, stressful hospital stay – I even wonder if in some subtle way, it helped influence me toward a successful outcome.

Making sense of the numbers: I've always appreciated Dr. Soiffer's directness with medical numbers. From mortality statistics to blood lab readings, he's always straightforward about sharing the metrics. As I've said before, I like the objectivity of numbers. But he also interprets the data, helping me distinguish between what's significant and what's not. He looks at trends as well as snapshots. He doesn't get too concerned about the inevitable little ups and downs – rather, he frames everything in the big picture perspective. I've seen the same thing in many of my other providers as they make sense of my various test readings and the like - I think that's a valuable doctoring trait.

Accessibility and responsiveness: Dr. Soiffer is a busy guy, and he certainly has a lot of high-stakes responsibilities on his plate. Even so, I've always been impressed how quickly he responds to emails and texts. His emails are usually short – once his entire reply to a question of mine consisted of the single word "no." In its own endearing way, that was eloquent! Way back when I was at home a few weeks after my transplant, I had a horrible stomach infection. I actually felt myself slipping away. As my condition worsened, Mary Ann and Soiffer were exchanging texts about my symptoms, temperature, and so forth. Finally, he texted her to "get him to the ER fast." That may have helped save my life. We later learned he was doing all this while at a Celtics game.

Clear visions of the future: Another attribute of good doctoring is providing the patient with a vision of the future. This can take many forms. For example, during the orientation I mentioned above, they gave us a tour of the radiation room where I'd receive my treatments - that helped lessen my anxiety about that frightening process. The nurse focused Mary Ann and me on steps we'd need to take *after* I got home from the hospital – that was valuable in more than just practical ways. In our various trips to the Emergency Room, we always found it calming and reassuring when the staff kept telling us what would come next. The most satisfying doctor visits all tend to end with a clear plan for the next steps. I think the common denominator with all these things is that a clear vision of the future helps fill in the void of uncertainty, and thus alleviates anxiety.

Laying out options: I've noticed a great attribute among several of my doctors: They present options, and discuss the pros and cons with me. A good example was my ear surgeon. After the skin graft he performed didn't take, he talked me through three options for the next step. He even drew little diagrams of each on the exam table paper – that was excellent! My eye doctor recently did a similar thing with possible remedies for my eye irritation – he involved me in the discussion, and together we laid out a strategy for Phase A, Phase B, and so forth. Dr. Soiffer and I often discuss options for adjusting my medications – he certainly takes the lead, but allows me to toss in my input. I think this helps the patient understand things better, and also feel more bought-in to the decision.

Translating medical terms into everyday language: I find it helpful when doctors translate complex medical terminology into simple language and images. A couple examples: I was struggling to understand part of a highly technical radiologist's report on my colonoscopy results – it seemed to be describing a particular after-effect on my colon from my radiation treatments years earlier. My family doctor clarified it by saying, "Oh, that's like a little pinch point." Got it! My lung doctor was interpreting my pulmonary test results, in particular my tendency to almost collapse after moderate exertion. He explained that each breath was piling up more and more CO_2 into my lungs, like "adding another pancake to the stack." That explained everything! It didn't necessarily make my breathing problems go away, but it sure helped to understand them. That in turn eased my frustration – one more example of the value of clear information.

A human, engaging manner: I've mentioned this so many times in my story, I don't think I need to elaborate too much here. I've always appreciated the doctors who engage on a human level. It can take many forms: a little personality, chit-chat, humor, or even just attentive body language. I'll never forget the time in the hospital when Dr. Soiffer said I was doing so well that I was "boring." That was beautiful! Or the time my dermatologist – who'd been a dancer before going to medical school – started doing ballet twirls right in the exam room! But an engaging manner is more than just a light-hearted moment here and there. It's about building rapport, fostering dialog, asking and answering questions, making the patient feel comfortable and involved in their treatment. I would guess that leads to better outcomes.

Preparation and focus: This incident may sound a bit contrary to the point above, but it showed another aspect of great doctoring: In one of our first meetings with the surgeon who would finally fix Mary Ann's ankle, he strode into the exam room right past us, and went immediately to the x-ray screen. My first impression was that seemed sort of brusque. But then he called us up to the screen and showed her x-rays, pointing out the ongoing problems with her ankle. Then he put up a diagram of his plan to fix it – it was neat, thorough, and impressive! The guy might not have had the warmest manner (at least at first), but he sure as hell did his homework. Rigorous preparation, total focus, pure competence. He ended up doing an amazing job saving Mary Ann's ankle, and she even got him to smile a few times.

Occasionally breaking the code of silence: This one might be on the controversial side. I'm not sure if there really is something called the "code of silence" among doctors – I just made it up. But I do know that many professions have a tendency to circle together and never criticize one of their own. Probably a good thing for the most part. But sometimes it is helpful to speak up. Soon after Mary Ann's first ankle surgery, her pain was so bad that she had to go to the Emergency Room. An orthopedic resident looked at her x-rays, closed the curtains around her bed, and whispered to us that her ankle had not been repaired well. A couple months later, after an unsuccessful second surgery, another orthopedic doc wasn't so subtle: He blurted out, "I get pissed when I see shoddy work like that!" We'll always appreciate how those two guys spoke up. Their ultimate purpose was to do what's best for the patient, and their candor probably ended up helping Mary Ann to walk again.

Acknowledging limitations: The doctor above who said he got pissed also demonstrated another admirable trait when we asked if he could repair Mary Ann's ankle. He said he'd be willing to team up with his colleagues and give it a try, but her ankle was so messed up it was outside their regular realm of expertise. He candidly said we'd be better off going to a trauma specialist at another hospital – a competing hospital! We appreciated his honesty, as well as what turned out to be a great referral. A similar example was the Mohs surgeon whose skin graft on my ear didn't take. First of all, he said that happened in 2% of his grafts – I found that a great use of statistics to provide context. Then I asked if he wanted to make a second attempt. He said he'd be willing to give it a shot, but my ear was now so disfigured that he felt a reconstructive specialist would be a better choice. I always appreciate when doctors (and others) are direct and honest about their limitations. It's interesting how so many of our bad doctoring experiences revolved around failure to do so.

Good point guard skills: In basketball, the point guard is the player who brings the ball up court and sets up the team's offense. A good point guard sees the whole play unfolding ahead, and knows when to pass the ball off to a teammate or take the shot him/herself. I think that's a good metaphor for a valuable trait we've experienced with some of our doctors: Knowing when to handle things yourself, and being comfortable (and well informed) making referrals and yielding to other providers. My family doctor in particular does a great job of this. So does my dermatologist. Unfortunately, we never found such a person with Mary Ann's ankle and knee injuries, and that led to a long, difficult orthopedic odyssey. With such a complex, disjointed web of healthcare options out there, having a trusty point guard to rely on is more essential than ever.

Overall, the vast majority of our doctor visits and provider encounters have been outstanding. Thanks to you all!

Many medicines besides drugs

I'd now like to share a few suggestions that Mary Ann and I have found helpful, even therapeutic, during our long healthcare journey. Let's call them "medicines." Most of these pertain to patients and caregivers, others to families and friends, some to providers, and even several for couples in general. It's a mixed bag of medicines. Help yourself to whatever you find of value - no prescription needed!

Taking charge of your care: It all starts with being proactive about getting check-ups in the first place. You might catch problems in time to fix them. I sure did. And if challenging conditions do arise, don't be a passive passenger - take charge of your care. This can take many forms: Do your homework; learn about your condition and treatment options; research various providers; network with others; make informed choices. Prepare for your doctor visits as if for a job interview. Write down your symptoms so you can give the doc a complete update; also write down your questions - otherwise you'll forget to ask. During the meeting, speak up; ask good questions; make sure you understand everything. Go with a partner if possible – two sets of ears are better than one. Managing your care is empowering - it gives you back a sense of control that the disease itself may have stripped away. It also leads to better decisions, and I think maybe even better outcomes.

Specific information: I've found specific information to be a valuable type of medicine. Whether in the form of numbers, dates, distinct options, specific action steps, or even clear language, information is an antidote to uncertainty. I've always found concrete information calming, even when it indicated "bad news." I'd take the clarity of bad news over the fog of uncertainty any day. Part of this should come from the doctoring side, as I've already mentioned in the Good Doctoring section. But patients and partners bear some responsibility, too. Seek out the specifics. Ask clarifying questions. Strive to walk away from each doctor encounter with clear explanations and action steps. Amidst the swirl of emotions and stress, specific information gives you something tangible to latch onto.

Avoiding overload: On the other hand, *too* much information can be harmful. In one of our early meetings at Dana Farber, the head transplant nurse gave us a huge 3-ring binder with all sorts of articles and resources about bone marrow transplants. At first it looked overwhelming. But she helped us focus on the most important parts, and encouraged us not to worry about the rest. That's great advice for people in the early stages of cancer, because your mind is craving information, and you're very susceptible to overload. At the same time, people tend to bombard you with all sorts of advice, books, articles, brochures, and referrals to every doctor or patient who ever had anything remotely to do with your situation. Don't get me wrong – it's all well-meaning. Just don't feel compelled to take it all in or follow every suggestion.

Milestones and benchmarks: You've probably noticed how often I've referred to various types of benchmarks and milestones. These include dates, year counts, holidays, elevations of peaks climbed, sports performance metrics, and so forth. I've grown to appreciate how these things give you goals to shoot for, and help track your progress. Holidays and anniversaries provide opportunities for reflection and insight. Just think of the special significance Halloween, Thanksgiving, and New Years have taken on for me. I guess it's all a way to create a little sense of order out of chaos. We're all on journeys of one sort or another, and specific milestones help mark and enrich our way.

Keeping good records: I've found it very helpful to document everything. Keep receipts of every medical expenditure from co-pays to parking fees. Track every mile driven. You'll be amazed how much you can deduct at tax time for medical expenses. This will also help if any insurance issues arise - good records are your best ally when dealing with the insurance companies. And maybe most important of all, meticulous record keeping gives you a "project" you can focus on, and a sense of at least something that you can control.

Humor: Throughout this journey, I've been blessed to have a partner with a great sense of humor. Neither of us is very good at telling canned jokes – if we did stand-up comedy, we'd certainly bomb. But somehow we seem to find the humor in the little situations around us. I'll always remember our laughter when the ER staff vacuumed the glass shards out of me after my moose collision; our playful caricatures of the endearing quirks of our health providers; Mary Ann's little dance moves on her crutches; her "Mr. No Ass" teasing of my shrinking physique, and so on. To this day, we still enjoy playful banter. We complete each other's jokes. We send silly texts and photos back and forth when we're separated by work travel. Maybe most therapeutic of all, we make fun of ourselves. Apparently, there's a lot of research out there confirming the tangible health benefits of laughter. I couldn't agree more. Humor has not only helped us cope through our many health challenges, but has also enriched our relationship overall. Humor might be the most potent medicine of all!

Accepting help: There's a lot of great medicine out there that we often fail to take advantage of. It comes from the generosity of others who offer their help. For some reason, we tend to say "no, thanks" a little too readily. Maybe this comes from a macho, "I-can-handle-it-myself" mindset; or maybe it's more of an "I-don't-want-to-be-a-burden" type of martyrdom. In any case, you're losing out in two ways: First of all - and I can't think of a more elegant way to say it - help can be helpful. Take advantage of it. During our most difficult periods, countless folks helped us out with rides, errands, meals, chores around the house, referrals, and all sorts of generous offers and kind gestures. They all made a difference. Secondly, it's not an imposition when you accept others' help. No, quite the opposite. You're honoring their generosity – you're actually giving *them* a gift! So when others ask "Is there anything I can do," take them at their word – come right out and ask for whatever you need. Everybody wins.

253

Respect for all your providers: I'll always remember the kindness my mother showed to her attendants during her long stay in the rehab center. This was in stark contrast to several other patients I overheard nearby, who sounded grouchy or rude. Over the years, several of my nurses and doctors have confided that some of their other patients were unpleasant to deal with. It makes me wonder why the heck anyone would not be nice to the people taking care of their health? Mary Ann and I have always tried to respect and connect with *all* our providers, especially the "lower level" staff. (I hate that phrase, but you know what I mean.) We ask questions about *them*, show some appreciation for the work they do, try to offer a compliment or some kind words when we can. As a result, we've had all sorts of interesting stories and feel-good moments. Hospitals and doctors' offices can be cold enough places with all their monitors and medical equipment and exam tables. A little human connection can warm up your encounters there, and maybe even give you some pleasant memories to take along on your journey.

The power of pets: I probably didn't stress enough in this story the amazing role our cats have played. Little Gizmo and Peng – they've been with us ever since our third date, and they're still going strong. They've been a constant source of amusement and joy and tenderness. They've kept us grounded during the tough times, and enriched our relationship overall. Every night around 3-4 am, I feel a light scratching on my arm - I lift the blanket and Gizmo crawls under and curls up with me. What a great little ritual! There's just something about animals. When Mary Ann and I encounter dogs on our walks, we both dissolve into babbling doggy-talk – it's almost like a surge of some happy drug running through our brains. I guess that's why they bring dogs into hospitals – apparently, they really do have some healing power. There's even research that says petting an animal lowers your blood pressure. Pets don't give you advice, or give you pep talks, or tell you how you should feel, or dump their own issues or judgments on you. They just give you pure, unadulterated, unconditional love - one of the most powerful medicines of all. Maybe we could all learn a few lessons from pets.

Letting people feel how they feel: The above point about pets reminds me of a bit of wisdom for friends and family members of cancer patients. It may run counter to our natural human impulses. I don't mean to disparage the attempts we all make to "cheer people up" or get them to "look on the bright side." That's all well-intended. But sometimes in the midst of the down moments, it's best just to let the patient (or caregiver or anyone else) feel how they feel, without trying to change their viewpoint or talk them into different emotions. Hold the advice, hold the remediation, hold the "Yes, but..." or "Well at least..." phrases for a while. There will soon be the right moment to start coaxing things back to the bright side. But it isn't now. Just listen, acknowledge, and support – no strings attached. That's one of the most helpful medicines you can offer.

Blanket kicking: Well this one definitely needs some explanation. It comes from a peculiar habit of our cat Gizmo when he sees the edge of a blanket pulled back or folded over. He lunges at it in full attack mode, flops onto his side, grabs the blanket with his forepaws, and ferociously kicks at it with his hind legs. We think he must be fantasizing about taking down a wildebeest on the Serengeti! But in reality, he's a little wimp who couldn't even dispatch a mouse. All that blanket kicking is just an overblown show of force, maybe some sort of outlet. Mary Ann and I have adopted the phrase "blanket kicking" to describe those instances where we each vent out a little stress or frustration or anger. It's become a very therapeutic coping mechanism along our way, allowing each other to let off a little steam now and then without getting too caught up in the emotion of the moment. Thanks, Giz!

Purpose: There's an old saying up here along the Maine coast that a boat deteriorates much faster when it sits idle in the harbor than when it's out in the open sea. I think there's some valuable wisdom there, especially for people going through long health struggles. While there's certainly a time for rest, I believe there's also danger in idleness. Physical limitations can spread quietly into other areas, like a stealthy creep, leading to inertia, stagnation, and more. From atrophying muscles to stalled career growth, I've come face to face a few times with the effects of my own inertia, and it's been terrifying. Fortunately, there's a good antidote: a sense of purpose. Purpose can take many forms, such as projects, goals, learning, creativity, mental stimulation, and any type of meaningful activity. It's all about striving, stretching, and moving onward.

Familiar comforts: At first glance, this part might seem to contradict the theme of the point above, but I feel "complement" is the more accurate word. In the midst of our fast-paced, ever-changing life over the years, Mary Ann and I have grown to appreciate the comforting little rituals we've developed at home. Examples include our morning coffee talks, regular treat times with the cats, Friday night glasses of wine, sprawling out with the Sunday paper, and so forth. Familiar routines give you a sense of stability and control - a calming antidote to the uncertainty and stress of medical challenges.

Good health insurance: Sorry for shifting the mood a bit here, but if we're talking about different kinds of medicines, good health insurance has to be one of them. Emphasis on the word "good." The emotional stress of poor coverage, or no coverage, or huge deductibles, or astronomical premiums, or vaguely defined coverage with lots of exceptions buried in fine print, can be far worse than the physical problems themselves. It all goes back to that awful nightmare of uncertainty I've mentioned so often. Mary Ann and I have gone through this at various times during our journey, and believe me, it's been brutal. The benefits of good health insurance are so much more than financial. A good plan gives you peace of mind, which is a powerful medicine in itself. It liberates you to go about the business of living the best life you can. I wish all our political leaders could grasp this, not only for individual Americans and families, but for the nation as a whole.

Exercise: I certainly don't want to end this list with the depressing topic of health insurance (especially the way it continues to be tossed about like a political football these days), so let me conclude with a couple more positive medicines. Wouldn't it be great if you could sort through every vitamin, supplement, diet, and self-help guide out there, searching for the very best of everything for a healthy body, mind, and spirit, and then distill it all down into one single super-pill? Well guess what? That pill already exists - and it's simple, cheap, and easily available to everyone. It's called exercise. Enough said on that.

Empathy: Finally, there's a medicine that underlies or interlinks many of the others I've already mentioned: plain old empathy. Empathy works in many directions. For example, empathy for the doctor struggling to keep up with an overloaded schedule; for the underappreciated efforts and sacrifices of the caregiver; for the awkwardness others feel when they struggle to find the right words to ask about your cancer; for the way the patient might not feel like "looking at the bright side" right now; or for the way others might not want to hear the details of your own medical issues right now. Empathy for the stresses and strains your partner might have bottled up inside; and empathy toward their different styles and strengths and ways of handling things. Empathy for the quiet burden the cancer survivor still carries after they're long past the critical period and everyone starts to move on. On a superficial level, you could say that empathy is a way to realize that it's not all about you. But ultimately, empathy really *is* about you – it enhances your interactions, deepens your relationships, and thus enriches your world.

So there you go. I hope you find some of the above medicines helpful. Let me know if you'd like to suggest any others, and we'll keep this conversation going. Thanks.

Part 12

UNEXPECTED
SIDE EFFECTS

*W*ell, it's been quite a journey. There are many ways to track how far we've come: Deep into year eight. 44,327 miles driven to medical appointments (almost twice around the planet Earth). Nearly a quarter-million dollars spent. Three homes, about to move into a fourth. More ups, downs, detours, and side roads than we ever could measure. An ever-lengthening book in search of a tidy ending.

Well I'm afraid that tidy ending is nowhere in sight – the long road onward continues. But now that I've finally finished the previous section about doctoring and medicines – the "helping" stuff I really wanted to get out there - I think it's a good time to wrap things up. So if you don't mind, I'd like to close with some personal reflections.

Have you ever been driving somewhere and you take a wrong turn, and at first you get all panicked and stressed out about being lost... but suddenly you stumble on a pleasant surprise? Maybe a quaint little store, or a beautiful vista, or a memorable encounter with a friendly stranger? An unexpected bonus that you never would have encountered if you hadn't gotten thrown off course?

Well cancer has certainly knocked my life off course. Mary Ann's, too. And we've sure had our share of frustration and stress as a result. But just like those pleasant surprises when you get lost on a road trip, I've picked up a few of my own along this medical journey. Let's call them unexpected side effects – the good kind.

I was reminded of this the other day at the eye doctor's, of all places. While most of my symptoms have been manageable lately, my eye problems have continued. Recently they flared up badly - swollen, red, painful, horrible looking, blurred vision, etc. So there I was at the eye doctor getting it checked out. As part of the exam, they gave me a vision test. I flunked. My eyes were so irritated that I could barely see the screen across the room, let alone read the letters.

But then I asked if I could try a little experiment. I put in some eye drops, tilted my head back, and closed my eyes for a while. When I re-opened them, I blinked my eyes in amazement - the screen was crystal clear, and I could read the next-to-bottom line. Turned out my distance vision was 20-20! That's better than it ever was before my leukemia. Within a few minutes, my eye irritation returned, and my vision got cloudy again. But that brief window of clarity revealed an amazing surprise: Despite years of dried out tear ducts and inflamed eye lids and irritated corneas, somehow my visual acuity, at least for distance, has actually improved! How's that for an unexpected side effect?

That got me thinking. It dawned on me that I've picked up many other surprising bonuses along the way. For example, way back in my pre-cancer years, when I was at the peak of my hiking-skiing-biking fitness, I had chronically high cholesterol. Never could shake it. But recently, despite all my problems with liver and digestion and weakened lungs and everything else, for some reason my cholesterol has improved. Go figure.

Same thing with my weight. I'm at an age when most guys are adding pounds and inches to their midsections. Not me. I still wear size 32 waist jeans. In fact, I probably could stand to add a few pounds. (Just ask my mother.) So every now and then, I can dive into some Ben and Jerry's or rich New England clam chowder without guilt.

Now as much as I love good ice cream, other unexpected benefits have been far more meaningful. One of the nicest has been the way my life has been enriched by so many great encounters with my healthcare providers. Countless stories that I never would have experienced otherwise. I've mentioned quite a few already. Let me add one more - one that has taken on renewed significance lately. You'll see why.

Way back during my hospital stay for my transplant, the head of my nursing team was a woman named Nejor. I'll always remember her kind, gracious manner – so calming during that time of anxiety and discomfort. We had great conversations, and Nejor shared her own amazing story. She grew up in East Africa amidst famine and civil war. As a young girl, she saw several relatives tortured and killed in front of her eyes. Her parents always stressed the importance of reading and learning as her ticket to a better life, and they taught her about this magical place called America – a land of safety and opportunity. She managed to flee, made it to New York, studied hard at school, enrolled in community college courses, kept learning...

...and now here she was at one of the top cancer hospitals in the US, leading the nursing team that helped save my life. I'll always remember the night of my transplant, the way Nejor calmly orchestrated the complex tasks among the team. And then when she came into the room cradling that pink bag of stem cells in the palms of her hands, and transfused new life into me, wow - I can't even think of words to describe how powerful that was.

And the thing is, Nejor was an immigrant. An immigrant with dark skin and a funny name and Muslim faith. By any reasonable measure, a success story about America at its best. Unfortunately, when I hear the ignorant nonsense about immigration that has infected our politics recently, I can only shake my head and sigh. But I'm glad my personal encounter with Nejor will live on far above all that. I'll always remain inspired by her story, and touched by the kind, competent way she took care of me.

That's just one of many such encounters I've been fortunate to have during my cancer journey. I think the broader "side effect" is that I've become more open to this type of connection overall, not just with medical staff but with folks in general. Mary Ann has, too. For some reason, we've each grown more likely to stop and connect with people whom we otherwise might have rushed past and barely noticed – especially those from outside our own little bubble.

On a related note, I think we've both become more compassionate. A bit softer in the heart. More deeply touched by the plight of the unfortunate. More likely to commit random gestures of kindness, like offering a compliment to a stranger, or giving a gift for no particular reason. Mary Ann in particular has been great about this. She keeps reminding me that every act doesn't always need a pragmatic purpose – just do something nice for the sake of doing something nice. We've made several decisions out of this spirit lately, and it feels great. I hope we keep it going.

Another meaningful side effect from this journey: Along with the surprising improvement in my long-distance vision, I think my vision inward has also sharpened. I've definitely become more introspective and self-aware. More humble, too. You get that way when you've been knocked down by cancer. I've learned things about myself, such as how I make decisions, how I cope with challenges, and how I act as a partner. I've become more aware of my little quirks. I've become more conscious of ruts, and more terrified of stagnation. Along with physical exercise and mental stimulation, I've realized how important it is to keep looking in the mirror and evolving as a person. Just writing this story has helped.

Come to think of it, the act of writing has been so therapeutic, maybe I should have included it in the "Many Medicines Besides Drugs" section. I'd highly recommend journaling or blogging or some type of writing to anyone going through a long health challenge.

And speaking of writing, even this book itself has been an unintended "side effect" of sorts - something that never would have happened if I hadn't gotten sick. I never in a million years thought I would ever write a book. And here I am, a few paragraphs away from finishing this one. I have no idea if it's any good, or if anybody will ever buy a copy, let alone find it helpful. I sure hope so, but I'm OK otherwise. I've spent several years laboring over this story, and I've finally gotten it to the point where it says what I wanted to say. To tell the truth, I'm proud of it, and that's good enough for me.

———◈———

Mary Ann and I often have great "what if" discussions looking back at the little twists and turns of history. For example, what if the wind shifted and the Spanish Armada won? What if Lee Harvey Oswald missed? What if a couple Supreme Court justices had ruled differently on those hanging chads in Florida? Huge movements in history have often hinged on little moments that could have gone either way. It's fascinating to speculate on how things would have turned out differently.

Same with our own journey. We've looked back and realized how life can change in an instant. A slip on an icy path, a blood count a few percentage points off, and life can veer off in a totally new direction. You get more appreciative of the fragility of it all, which makes you cherish each moment all the more. You learn not to take anything for granted.

You look back and ask yourself those "what if" questions about your own life: What if the moose plowed another three inches through my windshield? What if I never went in for that first blood test? What if we stuck with the first cancer hospital and waited six months to call them back? What if that kid at Syracuse University didn't notice the poster for bone marrow donor registration? What if Dr. Soiffer didn't return Mary Ann's text the night I was slipping away with my intestinal infection? What if we never got the referral to the trauma surgeon who finally repaired Mary Ann's mangled ankle? What if my Year-5 downturn wasn't somehow nudged off its downward slide?

You wonder about those little twists and turns. Were they just random quirks of circumstance? Or was there some other force at work?

You think back to that odd sensation you felt in Jerusalem when the warmth from the Western Wall spread from your palm up your arm and through your body, and gave you a sudden feeling of connectedness with a people across the world and throughout the centuries...

You wonder about that rare April rainbow that appeared briefly the morning after your father died, and the surprisingly comforting way it reassured you that he was at peace...

You think about that night seven weeks after your transplant when you were lying on the bed curled up in the fetal position, unable to lift your head or speak a word, your body ravaged by infection and burning with fever, your mind dancing with hallucinations, feeling yourself starting to let go and slide off to a warm peaceful place, and you faintly hear your wife's voice, muffled and distant as if from a far-off echo chamber, saying "get him to the ER right away," and then something takes hold of you like a gentle hand and sweeps you up off the bed, and you somehow find the strength to put on a pair of boots and grab your wife and mother by the arms and slog through the drifting snow and drive a car for the first time in months through a raging blizzard in the dark of night to the Emergency Room where the staff ends up saving your life... Where did that surge of energy come from?

It gets you thinking about another type of side effect. Something a little harder to put your finger on. Something you can feel, but you can't define. Something that doesn't quite fit into your logical, tangible, pragmatic view of everything. A sense that there's something else, something more...

Yes, this journey has sure taken me to places that I might never have visited otherwise.

I sometimes wonder if any of this had a hand in the most pivotal "what if" moment of all for me - a moment so infinitesimally tiny that you'd barely notice it, yet which changed my life forever. It was a fleeting microsecond way back in 2005, when I was searching on Match.com and mistakenly typed 200 miles into my search radius instead of the usual 100, and soon afterward that quirky profile from the blonde in Montreal popped onto my screen. Was that just a plain old random typo, or did some mysterious force nudge me to press the wrong key? I'll never know for sure. But whatever the cause, it opened up a whole new universe for me.

Though our wedding ceremony is a bit of a blur to me now, I do recall stumbling through our vows. I didn't give the words a lot of thought at the time – I was just concentrating on saying them right and holding the emotions in check. I imagine it was the same for Mary Ann.

Recently I decided to look back and check what we actually said during those vows. So I pulled out a manila folder labeled "Wedding" that had been tucked away in the back of our file cabinet for many years. As I rifled through the folder, I came across our marriage license, invitation, reception menu, and other memorabilia – they all brought back warm memories. Then I pulled out a copy of our vows, which the Justice of the Peace had printed out for us on a nice piece of parchment. I started reading, and sure enough, there it was – the phrase I was wondering about, the phrase that stopped me in my tracks: "…in sickness and in health…"

I felt a little shudder go through me. Who could have imagined how that phrase would take on such meaning a mere ten months after the ceremony. And how powerfully it would continue to resonate throughout the years, right down to the present day. Well as for me, the resonance from that phrase – from that promise we made to each other - leads to one more unexpected side effect, maybe the unlikeliest of all: A sense that in some crazy way, taking care of each other through this odyssey has deepened our bond, enriched our life, and taken us to whole new realms.

My sweets, I can only hope you feel the same way.

So let me turn directly to you - there's something I want to tell you about this book. Yes, I wrote it with several different purposes in mind. But one stands above the rest. There are 89,571 words in this story, and every one of them is there for one ultimate goal: To thank you from the bottom of my heart for standing by me during this journey, inspiring me to struggle on when things got tough, and filling my life - and my soul - with more joy and wonder, and a deeper, richer love, than I ever dreamed anyone could experience.

Take my hand, sweets, and let's keep on strolling down that long road together...

CPSIA information can be obtained
at www.ICGtesting.com
Printed in the USA
JSHW011144040623
42627JS00004B/43